Keeping the Faith in Late Life

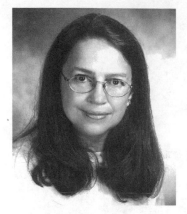
Susan A. Eisenhandler, PhD, is a professor of sociology at the University of Connecticut. Her qualitative research on age and identity has focused on understanding the meaning and value of interaction and social engagement among community-dwelling older adults. She and the late Gene Thomas, a UCONN colleague, collaborated on research and writing projects, including two books, *Aging and the Religious Dimension* and *Religion, Belief, and Spirituality in Late Life* (Springer Publishing Company, 1999). In addition, Dr. Eisenhandler has published scholarly articles that explore the definitions of self and situation that older adults invoke in everyday experiences. Dr. Eisenhandler is an active member of several community and professional organizations and has received grants to create and to facilitate community-based literature programs for older adults.

Keeping the Faith in Late Life

Susan A. Eisenhandler, PhD

Springer Publishing Company

Permissions
Excerpts from "Courage" and "Welcome Morning" from *The Awful Rowing Toward God* by Anne Sexton. Copyright © 1975 by Loring Conant, Jr., executor of the Estate of Anne Sexton. Reprinted by permission of Houghton Mifflin Company. All rights reserved.

Original art for frontispiece by Lucy Rose Fischer.

In order to protect privacy and maintain confidentiality, pseudonyms have been substituted for the real names of people who participated in the study. Likewise, their community or place of residence appears in the form of a pseudonym.

Springer Publishing Company, Inc.
536 Broadway
New York, NY 10012-3955

Acquisitions Editor: Helvi Gold
Production Editor: Sara Yoo
Cover design by Joanne Honigman

03 04 05 06 07/5 4 3 2 1

Library of Congress Cataloging-in-Publications Data

Eisenhandler, Susan A.
  Keeping the faith in late life / Susan A. Eisenhandler.
    p. cm.
  Includes bibliographical references and index.
  ISBN 0-8261-1775-9
  1. Aged—Religious life.   2. Aging—Religious aspects.   3. Aged—Religious life—Connecticut.   I. Title.
  BL625.4 .E35 2003
  306.6'084'6—dc21   2002036658

Printed in the United States of America by Sheridan Books.

To Jon Eisenhandler
and other gentle readers

Probe me, O God, and know my heart;
Try me, and know my thoughts;
See if my way is crooked,
And lead me in the way of old.

Psalm 139, Verses 23 and 24

This psalm had special meaning for two people in the study who called it a "favorite." The verses are taken from a Bible kept at home by one person.

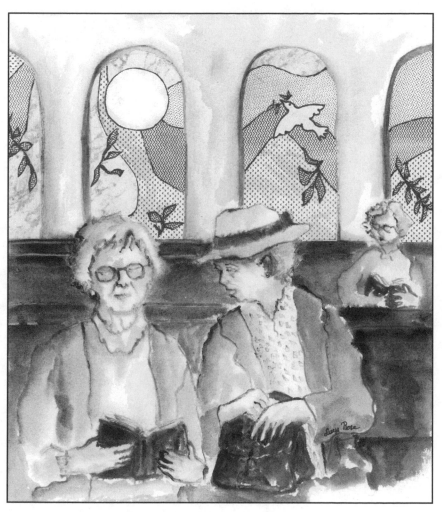

Frontispiece by Lucy Rose Fischer

Contents

Foreword

THAT OLD TIME RELIGION: IS IT GOOD ENOUGH FOR ME?

A memorable film titled "The Gods Must Be Crazy" tells a comic tale based on a familiar theme in anthropology: namely, surprise on the part of an isolated tribe when they stumble on the ways of modern civilization. In *Keeping the Faith* sociologist Susan Eisenhandler has accomplished a similar startling discovery: namely, Eisenhandler has found a "tribe" of modern Americans who *don't* move every three years, who *don't* get divorced or find new jobs, and above all, who *don't* change their religion or sign up for psychotherapy or some variety of New Age philosophy. And who is this remarkable tribe? None other than descendants of our New England ancestors, residents of Connecticut, that "State of steady habits." These members of the tribe are respondents in Eisenhandler's sample, the ones who participated in her study of religious experience in later life.

As a skilled qualitative researcher Eisenhandler is able to convey her story with some depth and in detail. A familiar hymn insists that "That old-time religion is good enough for me" and Eisenhandler's respondents tell us that the old-time religion is good enough for them, too. Here indeed is the overriding conclusion of this book: Religion remains a bulwark of meaning for later life. This conclusion is an important message for a 21st century world which routinely tells itself that "the only thing that's constant is change itself." Yet sociologists, from Durkheim to the present, are looking for constancy as well as change. They look for deep structures, patterns of social dynamics that endure and offer an explanation for the behavior we find around us, including religion in old age. The findings in Eisenhandler's book confirm the role of religion as a "bedrock" of later life. Her sample consisted entirely of people with substantial religious experience during childhood or youth, so their "bedrock socialization" reaches back to childhood and has continued in a lifelong pattern of religious affiliation and participation. The pattern remains even where subjective faith takes on different forms over the years. "Still faithful after all these years" is an apt summary for this entire volume.

A central finding of this book is the reverberating impact of childhood over the life course. The folkways of faith established in our early years tend to endure. "Religion is something you carry with you" or "Religion is a habit" were common responses here. Despite shifts in gender roles, innovations in liturgy, and changes in the broader culture, respondents in this study still "keep the faith." Like a strong tree solidly anchored in the earth, they may bend in the wind but they retain their sturdy roots in the soil of ancestral piety.

Participants in Eisenhandler's sample were born and came of age before W.W. II. They grew up at a time when religion was not a matter of individual choice or decision. Whether living independently or in a long-term care setting, older adults in this study were inclined to "keep the faith" by adapting or reinterpreting elements of religion that might appear problematic or troubling at times, such as life after death or the existence of multiple coexisting faith traditions (can they all be true?) Eisenhandler documents the ways her respondents "bend" to shifting religious practices: for example, changes in ritual in the main-line churches.

Eisenhandler's sample is characterized by powerful geographic and residential stability: her respondents all tend to stay in the same place. Faith, then, is understood as a sense of belonging, more powerful perhaps than specific doctrinal beliefs about God. Even doubters, or near-atheists, felt the social obligations of their congregational community.

Despite the emphasis on community, Eisenhandler's research also confirms the importance of prayer in later life. Daily prayer is the most often mentioned instance of religious behavior among older people. But even the practice of prayer, this most important folkway of late-life religion, turns out to be a multifaceted phenomenon. For example, some respondents in this study use standard prayers, while others made up their own prayers, whether of gratitude, praise or petition. Prayer remains a powerful way of creating and sustaining meaning and purpose in later life.

And who exactly are these people praying to? Eisenhandler shows that God is generally understood by her respondents in figurative or symbolic terms: as a divine "Other" who listens to prayer. This is not "contemplative" prayer, as the mystical tradition would frame it: as, for instance, in the great medieval treatise *The Cloud of Unknowing*. Indeed, the pattern of prayer found by Eisenhandler is what she terms *reflexive* and it is carried on through familiar forms from childhood. Even when its vocabulary is limited, this form of prayer is meditative and subjectively meaningful. It is not "magical" in purpose nor is it prayer that is self-interested in any narrow instrumental sense. The enduring power of early socialization is impressive, even when it does not seem to flower into introspection or reflection.

This book considers an important problem raised by the demography of religious participation: namely, the graying of American religion. Older people, at least in mainline churches, are by far the largest proportion of people sitting in the pews. Yet older folks are too often taken for granted by clergy: what Eisenhandler labels a sort of "benign neglect" on the part of religious leaders. This pattern is well-known. National gerontological groups have long pointed to neglect of aging on the part of organized religion. Older people themselves are "keeping the faith" but the same cannot be said of religious leaders, who are in the same state of denial as other opinion leaders.

Does firmness and constancy of religious habits preclude growth or change? The question is intriguing for those concerned with spiritual development over the life course. Eisenhandler quotes one respondent as saying "To a good degree that sometimes the more questions you have, then maybe the more you get unstable, you're not as firm in beliefs," and she goes on to say that "that never happened to me." Firmness of faith sounds admirable. But spiritual growth may demand something more. Contrast the "Don't ask questions" response with the remark by Thomas Merton, who once remarked that we do not prayer properly because we do not doubt sufficiently.

Eisenhandler found a profoundly social experience of religion in her sample, but she also found appreciation of the natural world as an important complement to institutionalized religion. She did not find in her sample much of what could be called mystical experience or a sense of divine presence, in contrast to Jeffrey Levin, who found many experiences of the paranormal among respondents to a national survey sample about aging and religious practice. Eisenhandler notes that respondents in her sample seemed to have a very different religious sensibility than, say, Baby Boomers with their pursuit of what Wade Clark Roof has termed "the spiritual marketplace."

The solidity and stability of these self-reports raise questions about our developmental ideas about religion: for instance, as expounded by

James Fowler in his idea of "stages of faith." Eisenhandler for the most part did not find people moving toward higher stages. Nor did she find what Robert Atchley called "everyday mysticism." However, Eisenhandler did find some examples of what Joan Erikson and later Lars Tornstam have called "gero-transcendence." Eisenhandler found a tendency, at least among a minority, toward increased interiority in later life, a trend documented by the original Kansas City Studies that first gave rise to the much-disputed idea of disengagement. For these "inner-directed" respondents Eisenhandler found a measure of positive disengagement that stands in contrast both to the power of social habits and the celebration of activity so pronounced among contemporary American images of a good old age.

The news here is that outer stability and inner growth can coexist. In her probing interviews, Eisenhandler shows how it is possible to practice the familiar "faith of our fathers" but with deeper levels of realization or understanding. For example, 85-year old Jack, one of the oldest men in Eisenhandler's sample, finds himself pondering the relationship between religious faith and the findings of physics and astronomy: the sort of reflection that is honored in the Templeton Prize for Religion. Similarly, 90-year-old Ellen has become more detached from external religious practice but is deepening her understanding of faith in other ways, thus displaying the tolerance Fowler would identify with higher levels of spiritual development.

In broad terms, Eisenhandler finds two large "varieties of religious experience" among her respondents. She distinguishes between reflexive (habitual) and reflective (meditative) forms of faith. What she finds, overwhelmingly, is the enduring power of folkways, or religious practices that direct people into specific behavior without requiring any deeper thought. The second dimension, or reflective faith, amounts to "stretching the soul" or moving beyond habitual patterns into a more mature form of faith.

Another intriguing feature of this sample is age segregation or age concentration. The respondents in Eisenhandler's sample constitute a "time capsule" that speaks to us with the voice of say, Middletown, U.S.A., in 1938. Indeed, Eisenhandler's sample, as she herself says at one point, almost seems to mimic traditional societies. It is on just this point that we may offer some reflections on the role of so-called "traditional" religion and even suggest some other ways of interpreting Eisenhandler's findings.

Traditional religion the world over has included forms that fit more or less into Eisenhandler's distinction between reflexive and reflective faith: namely, exoteric and esoteric traditions. In Tibetan Buddhism, for instance, there is a popular folk religion reflected in multiple deities and magical practices. Popular religion coexists with a refined form of Buddhist meditation and cosmopolitan awareness maintained to this day by the Dalai Lama. Similarly, Christianity ranges from fundamentalist forms of literal understanding to the varieties of contemplative prayer found among the Desert Fathers as well as in Saint Theresa or Thomas Merton in our own time. The same distinction between exoteric and esoteric religion can be found in Hindu, Islamic and other faith traditions. On the one side, is the emphasis on law, ritual, and literalism; on the other side, a deepening awareness of transpersonal reality.

The esoteric and exoteric forms of religion need not be in conflict, except when clergy or social authorities find themselves threatened by personal forms of spirituality. In Sufi, Zen and yoga traditions we see that popular and esoteric religion coexist and reinforce each other. But esoteric forms of faith are not matters of individual idiosyncrasy: they are organized forms of social practice, with their own rules of socialization, inter-generational transmission, and schemes for interpreting reality. The difference between exoteric and esoteric, in other words, is *not* simply reducible to a difference between conformity versus individualism. Alfred North Whitehead once remarked that religion is what individuals do with their aloneness. Eisenhandler notes that many people in her study commented that "with God you are never alone." The paradox is this: what we do with our aloneness we don't accomplish in isolation. Therein lies the whole logic of a monastery, whether Christian or Zen, and also of tertiary religious orders inspired by the patterns of socialization that reach beyond the cloister. The paradox is that we need to be socialized to learn to be alone with ourselves, and this learning may itself be the greatest gift of age.

Eisenhandler's study permits us to see the religion of later life today in longitudinal terms. It is both the product of conditions of conformity paramount in the 1940s and 1950s, and also of the religious diversity that has become more pronounced by the end of the 20th century. Other sociologists have reflected on this historical process. For instance, in *After Heaven: Spirituality in American Since the 1950s*, sociologist Robert Wuthnow draws a distinction between what he calls the spirituality of *dwelling* and the spirituality of *seeking*. The spirituality of dwelling belongs in houses of worship, in denominations, and in local neighborhoods influential during the 1950s. But by the 1960s, Wuthnow argues, we saw the rise of a spirituality of seeking, which led people to venture outside established religion in exploring a more authentic self. This polarity between dwelling and seeking finds its echo in Eisenhandler's distinction between reflexive and reflective faith traditions among her respondents.

But the point is that there is something limited about this dichotomy itself, a point which Wuthnow himself recognizes. Do we really have to choose between, say, conformist suburban church-going, on the one hand, or eclectic New Age inspiration, on the other? How do we bring together the spirituality of dwelling and seeking? How do we reconcile reflexive and reflective forms of faith? Eisenhandler recognizes that her "New England tribe" is waiting for answers to this dilemma. Wuthnow believes there are hopeful signs of resurgent interest in traditional spiritual disciplines, disciplines which acknowledge our encounter with the sacred (e.g., near-death experiences) while invoking practices that could help ground our sense of an inner, more authentic self.

This grounding will *not* be found in the endless "seeking" of today's "New American Spirituality," an impatient sensibility that often resembles channel surfing for the spirit. On the contrary, traditional teachings, as I have argued in *The Five Stages of the Soul*, involve a measure of commitment to a single path explored in depth. As Kierkegaard put it, purity of heart means to will one thing. Thus, commitment and exclusiveness can be consistent with tolerance, which is certainly a much-needed virtue in our current global environment. But respondents in Eisenhandler's sample understood this point when they themselves said "I'm not a fanatic but . . . " and then went on to speak about the importance of commitment to religion in their own lives. The Sufi aphorism put it this way: A garden has many gates but you can only enter the garden by going through a single gate at a time. The respondents in Eisenhandler's sample would probably agree, even if they had never heard of Sufism. That's what it means to "keep the faith."

But have today's older adults also been told about this garden which they are invited to enter on the other side of the gate? Eisenhandler fears they have not been so informed, and there lies her (implicit) critique of contemporary religious institutions. We need guidance, even socialization, to move toward the inner life of spirituality. Those who keep the faith, graying members of our congregations, are hungry for spiritual food but their leaders are not feeding them. Or perhaps, like Atchley's "everyday mystics," these old New England souls are already finding spiritual food growing right in their own gardens, in their own backyard. The great merit of Eisenhandler's research is that it turns our gaze in the direction of this garden and permits us to see in new ways the religious sensibility of old age.

HARRY R. MOODY

Preface

HOW THE STUDY EVOLVED

From participant observation as a driver of senior center vans to work as a teacher and facilitator in various community-based educational programs for older adults, and as a social gerontologist doing research on identity and late life, I have been fortunate to have played an active role in varied settings where reading, thinking, and discussion offered older adults possibilities for "significant being." I have met wonderful people in all of these settings, colleagues and older adults who made important contributions to the research studies and the work that was completed. Many of them are long since departed now, as is the case of at least two people from this recent community study.

As I formulated some new ideas about how to examine religious behavior and its role in daily life, it seemed a logical extension to expand my proverbial backyard from the greater Naugatuck Valley, where I am a professor of sociology for the University of Connecticut at its Waterbury campus, to include other rural, suburban, and urban communities in the state. It also appeared to be a propitious time to follow up on a suggestion tendered by a colleague in social gerontology, Jay Gubrium, who had recommended that I include interviews with older adults in long-term care facilities. I had not interviewed or completed research in nursing homes before, and it seemed to me that it was indeed time to enter the places where older adults are likely to face special circumstances when practicing or following their faith.

Moreover, the evolution of this research project has another source— the sociology of religion. My abiding interest in religion goes back to some research I did on ethnicity and religion for Bill Newman (it was as an undergraduate research assistant on one of his projects that I was introduced to open-ended questions and the fact that both religion and ethnicity defy easy categorization and have very blurry lines). This early interest was followed up some years later in a presentation, "The

Relationship Between Age and Religiosity: A Reappraisal," my husband, Jon, and I gave based on Gallup's 1978 poll "The Churched and Unchurched," to a 1980 meeting of the Society for the Scientific Study of Religion. That work emerged separately from other analyses we completed with Clark Roof during some of our graduate work in sociology at the University of Massachusetts. This qualitative study on religion grew from these earlier experiences and projects and in such a way that many lines of thought even now continue to evolve.

WHAT THE BOOK DRAWS TOGETHER ABOUT FAITH AMONG OLDER ADULTS

When I first conceived the fieldwork that provides the basis of this study, my goal was to see the world through the eyes of my respondents in order to get beyond the comfortable world where I defined the questions and circumscribed the answers. To this end, I asked people to give voice to their understanding of religion and how it fits into their world as their life draws to a close. While I should not have been surprised, the breadth of response intrigued me. There were people for whom religion provided the heartfelt core of their life. For others, religion was a social practice supported out of habit or obligation.

My fieldwork took place over the period of a year. In the course of the work I sat with each of my respondents for several hours. I asked general questions and then allowed them to frame their responses. We explored issues relating to religion and how they saw it fitting into their life, what they gave to it, and what they took from it. This book will be valuable to all students of religion and the life course who wish to understand some of the ways in which older adults experience and practice faith, for it contains the views, words, and responses of those older adults.

More pragmatically and with the thought of encouraging both observational fieldwork and face-to-face interviewing as an integral part of undergraduate and graduate studies, I believe professors will find the book useful as a text for students in general social science courses and in more substantively focused courses in social gerontology, psychology, sociology, or religious studies. The book may work particularly well in courses where students are asked to formulate specific qualitative research projects and exercises, or in classes that seek a coordinated project to bring to fruition during a semester. Sample questions included in the appendix are illustrative of some topics and issues that students may find helpful as examples to explore or to replicate in individual or group work.

The strengths of qualitative work and the reasons that it is well suited to research in human science are other themes that speak to teachers and students. There is good material here for class discussions worth holding about the heuristic and analytic dimensions of research and the relationship between what is uncovered in the field and how it supports or challenges other research. The book provides a springboard into the nature of interdisciplinary approaches and perspectives as they relate to the creation of knowledge and the application of that knowledge to situations in the everyday worlds where all of us reside.

Most of all I see the study as a very real way for educators of all stripes to remind and encourage students and other professionals to ask older adults about their experiences by getting out into the social worlds we often only observe from great distances. Students may discover that some features of a systematic research process are not at all beyond their efforts, and may become engaged in learning how to ask questions, listen, and how to understand what life means to people by talking with them. This strikes me as a good sound step to take in learning more about the research process and about the social worlds surrounding people most of whom hope to become older adults one day in the future.

From two opposite roles and perspectives in the research dynamic—that of the researcher and that of the research participant—the approach of qualitative research as a process and as a method of inquiry works well to open up discussion about religious matters and late life. The act of agreeing to open oneself to background questions as well as to questions about faith, and the act of seeking people willing to answer questions, are themselves processes of trust and faith as well as a rational set of objective explanations and lines of reasoning that are scientific or systematic and focused on research.

The chapters are organized to move readers through the central patterns of faith in the lives of older adults as those patterns were expressed and disclosed from their own words in the interviews. Chapter 1 is an overview of the theoretical and methodological points that guided the research and became the backdrop for understanding the experiences people described about faith. Chapter 2 discusses the accounts people gave of how religion and faith were instilled in their lives. Though childhood experiences and active participation by mothers laid the foundation for most elders, socialization to religion is also a collective or generational experience that is substantially different from that of younger cohorts. Chapters 3 and 4 take up the most significant themes and features of religion in late life—the folkways of faith, the customary ways that older adults pray, and the other ways that religion is practiced. Attendance and membership are not the most important folkways of faith for older adults, but prayer is crucial. Chapter 5 takes us to the thoughtful arena of musings, doubts, and questions of what I call a "grown-up" faith. Life and aging challenge many of the fundamental tenets of faith and people described many areas where their own interpretations and behaviors had changed. Chapter 6 considers the social setting of nursing homes and the special situations that affect the practice of faith among elders living in those settings. The dimensions of space and of autonomy are significant and the practice of prayer again emerges as crucial for involvement in religion. Chapter 7 raises the question that flows directly from the words of older adults who depicted their faith as largely reflexive, something taken for granted and an activity of habituation—can there be a reflective faith? Is it possible or necessary for the spirit and the sacred to move beyond a steady and steadfast religiosity?

Finding out about social scientific reality hinges on the basic elements of human interaction, listening and talking with people, understanding what is meaningful to them as individuals and for the group as a whole, hearing the themes that emerge from the voices of people. At the close of the interview, elders nearly always made the impromptu remark that they hoped they had given me "something useful" for the study, something that was worthwhile for others to consider about religion in late life. I hope, in short, that this book is something useful and that you will use it to stimulate fieldwork and interviewing especially with and among older adults.

Acknowledgments

There were many people who willingly and graciously lent a hand with a variety of tasks associated with planning and conducting the study, and with transforming hours of conversation and thoughts into the writing that appears here in the form of a book. First and foremost, I wish to thank the forty-six older adults who were interviewed and whose lives and thoughts are the rich material for this discussion of keeping the faith. In order to safeguard their privacy, their real names are covered by pseudonyms. I offer them the deepest appreciation for making me and my tape recorder welcome in their homes and for the thought they gave to the questions and to the interview process.

Other people assisted me in the process of finding interviewees. They nominated or referred people for the study. This help was essential to the fieldwork that brought researcher and older adults together for interviews in communities or long-term care facilities. In order to preserve the privacy of these study participants, I cannot thank each person who assisted in the nomination process by name. Similarly, I wish to thank the people I interviewed during the course of the study who provided religious or devotional programs to older adults. Though I cannot expressly include all of these people by naming each one, I thank each of them and all of them for their generous efforts and invaluable assistance.

Others who lent assistance that may be acknowledged explicitly include the fine staff members of the campus library, Sheila Lafferty, Janet Swift, and Susan Thebarge. I especially wish to thank Sheila for the professional help and resourcefulness she displayed in tracking down myriad details and sources that researchers always need and quite often cannot locate when left to their own devices. I also thank Maria Vega for the bibliographic work she completed for the project and for the simultaneous translation she provided in the interview process. Others who were part of the circle of the study by virtue of offering helpful comments and collegial suggestions include: Judith Baker, Michael Blumenthal, Helen Raisz, and Sister Marian Slezak.

I also extend my thanks to those who provided partial funding for expenses related to transcribing the many hours of tapes from the interviews: The University of Connecticut Research Foundation and the Consortium for Gerontological Education both provided support for these services. I also thank the Department of Sociology for the permission fee support it provided. In addition, I thank the Oral History Center at the University of Connecticut for the equipment loan of a top-of-the-line recorder, easily the best I've ever used in fieldwork. I also appreciate the quality of work completed by the transcriptionists working for Tapescribe under the deft supervision of Martha McCormick.

This leads to my final word of acknowledgment, to the person there for all the steps along the way, thank you, Jon.

CHAPTER ONE

Introduction: Faith as a Feature of Identity and of Late Life: The Theoretical and Methodological Context of the Study

> *"The love of God can keep you from bein' so awful lonesome sometimes too when you are settin' in a house by yourself thinkin' of the things that's tuk place in your life."*
> —Kate Brumby (Federal Writers' Project, 1975, p. 159)

INTRODUCTION

Keeping the Faith in Late Life is a book that describes and analyzes qualitative interviews gathered from women and men, sixty years old or older, who imparted their thoughts about the value and meaning of religion in their lives. The book is a distillation of many themes that people talked about, and traces religious folkways that surround and inform the practice of faith among older adults. It is a sociological narrative of religious belief and behavior that have been sustained and sometimes changed over the course of life and the process of growing old.

The collaborative work that the late Gene Thomas and I completed; that is, two edited volumes on the relationship between religion and aging, *Aging and the Religious Dimension* (1994) and *Religion, Belief, and Spirituality in Late Life* (1999), as well as my independent qualitative research into the relationship between old age and identity, were the foundations for the study and this book. With its 46 interviews of older adults, observational work, and interviews with people who provided programs to meet religious needs, programs that foster what Rabbi

1

Heschel once called "significant being" (1981, p. 38), the study adds another level to the analysis and discussion of meaning and identity in late life and to an appreciation for the various ways that religion is woven into the lives of older adults. It is a sociological record of the folkways of faith among a group of contemporary elders.

Unlike my colleagues in anthropology who often study esoteric and exceptional groups in their fieldwork, as a sociologist I aim to understand the characteristics of people or social actors who are an integral yet typical or ordinary part of the social worlds that are the nexus of culture and society. Connecticut, tagged for at least two centuries as "the land of steady habits," (Mathews, 1951, p. 954) is neither synonymous with nor to be confused with the esoteric. The 169 towns and cities of the state have become an almost seamless suburban milieu set off by occasional rural villages and towns and highlighted by relatively small-sized urban pockets (each of the state's five largest cities has less than 200,000 residents). The state provides a typical social backdrop for living and aging in contemporary America and qualifies as a satisfactory and fairly representative setting for the qualitative study of religious belief and behavior in late life. The thoughts and responses of older adults depicted here provide a window into the social reality and experiences of older adults across similar communities.

In terms of social gerontology, specifically the ways in which aging and faith are connected to the individual's sense of self-identity, this book examines personal engagement with religion, the role of socialization in retaining faith in late life, and the extent to which older adults participate in religious behavior and find religious beliefs relevant to their present life. As Kate Brumby disclosed decades ago in her remarks to an interviewer from the Federal Writers' project, "the love of God" is often a transcendent link that staves off loneliness in late life. Her view leads to questions about the role of religion for elders in the present. Do older adults today find such good company in the sacred or avail themselves of it? What social behavior is consonant with the recognition of having such a tie, of keeping faith as part of life? Other questions that were at the core of the research project were: What role does faith play in coming to terms with the many changes posed in late life? Does old age as a prelude to finitude stimulate a religious impulse toward life or a greater reflectiveness about one's life? How does the immediate social setting of place, living independently in the community as contrasted with living in a long-term care facility, influence the practice of faith? Is religion an anchor for the self-identity of older adults? In what ways does religion orient and integrate the older person into a larger social world? Where and how do people improvise or respond to features of religion that present obstacles to facing life instead of helping them face life's dilemmas? What happens when attendance and participation are no longer viable routes for religious practice?

The book synthesizes material educed from questions that were asked of everyone, and from questions that arose from unique characteristics of the people in the study and from their thoughts, musings, and doubts about religion and the folkways of faith. In the end, the content was shaped as much by the human participants and dynamic processes that underlie qualitative research as by the theoretical concepts and interview guide that directed the formal research project. This is a key strength of qualitative methodology and befits investigations that are not centered on testing theory or collecting uniform data for statistical extrapolations, projections, or profiles. Rather the methodology takes us to the field to draw together responses of those who are living and aging in the social contexts of interest, and to place these understandings of life in a broader framework. The resulting analysis creates a kind of bas-relief composed of figures, individuals, whose lives emerge separately but as a part of the backdrop. When viewed from a greater distance, the figures stand out from the background of culture and society; the patterns of religion and faith for individuals and for the group emerge for the whole.

The study and book are best understood as fitting within the long-standing tradition of qualitative works that evoke and illustrate dimensions of the interplay between social structure and individual, even as those studies and this one hold no brief for testing specific hypotheses. This field and community study of religion in late life is centered in that tradition, a place where researchers scan carefully and methodically to observe the ordinary environs, and perhaps every so often, to glimpse a rare bird captured up close for a moment within the lens of binoculars, or in this case, captured on tape and in transcription.

THE THEORETICAL LENS FOR THE STUDY: IDENTITY, MEANING, FOLKWAYS

This study makes use of three theoretical constructs derived from different disciplinary perspectives as ways to orient the research questions and as ways to discuss the patterns that emerge from the details and examples people relayed about religion in everyday life. The constructs, meaning, identity, and folkways are also sensitizing ones for the reader— they inform readers about the kind of discourse and analytic framework that shapes the research, and the framework used to make sense of what was found in the field research. This chapter is, in part, intended to give some sense of how these constructs, particularly identity and meaning (folkways are directly addressed in a later chapter) helped to guide the thinking for the project. The study was not designed to test or to build theory in a direct fashion as might be the case in more positivistic endeavors. Nonetheless, this trinity of theoretical constructs was used to formulate the study and to reflect on material gathered in the field. With this in mind, we turn to a brief discussion of the way identity is conceived and the fit between this conception and the use of qualitative research to explore it.

IDENTITY

It was William James who first distinguished between the "discriminated" aspects of identity, the I and the me, at the same time that he connected and subsumed both within the unitary self, a dynamic entity, capable of knowing and being known. Indeed, James pointed the way to a concept of self that departed from two competing but rather confining perspectives—the intrapsychic system of Freud and the metaphysics of religion. By centering his concern for self-awareness in the formation and maintenance of different components of the "me," the material, social, and spiritual dimensions, James (1929) forged a pathway whose destination was the account of how the responses of others influence the individual's sense of self. James's idea (1963, p. 169) that "Properly speaking, a man has as many social selves as there are individuals who recognize him and carry an image of him in their mind," was an attempt to move theories of self and identity out of the rigid confines imposed by psychoanalysis and religion. His work was pivotal in framing the self as social.

The work of analyzing relationships between individual and group— how individuals internalized norms of the group or donned a sociocultural wrapping for self and identity, while they simultaneously achieved some measure of independent thought and action; what mechanisms of social control enhanced the individual's solidarity with the group;

and the ways in which some individuals and groups accrued greater rewards for belonging while other individuals and groups did not— became the primary concerns and questions for early sociologists to pose. The symbolic interactionists articulated a theory of human behavior that focused on the meanings and interpretations given to social reality by the individual (Mead, 1964; Thomas & Znaniecki, 1958). The way to tap into these meanings and interpretations was summed up by Herbert Blumer (1969, p. 145). "Insofar as sociologists or students of human society are concerned with the behavior of acting units, the position of symbolic interaction requires the student to catch the process of interpretation through which they construct their actions."

This study of religious engagement captures the interpretation and action of acting units, here, individuals who are older adults, in the accounts and stories they tell about how they act with respect to religious beliefs and what they do to maintain their ties to others and to their God. Insofar as social science can capture moments of the processes inherent in self-indication and the formulation of meaning, conversations and interviews open a way to hearing, observing, and understanding those processes. Focused interviews permit the give-and-take of conversation to work through retrospective, contemporary, and prospective time frames for the topic of faith and daily life. Methodologically the social form and some of the salient contents of identity are expressed in the conversational flow of words, images, and ideas as well as in the interaction of the interview itself.

Identity Defined as Social Location

Central to the project is the conception of identity as the self that is constructed in the dynamic process of engagement and interaction between individual and others in various social worlds across a lifetime. A classic interactionist method of capturing identity revolves around the patterns and qualities evident in answers to the questions: Who am I? Who are you? People respond to these questions by pointing to, and in other ways naming and describing the elements of self and identity that are salient to them. In responding to these questions and in elaborating on their lives, people also reveal the folkways, customary ways of doing things, as well as the norms, guidelines to behavior, that they follow in interacting with others and in moving through social worlds every day. Thus, talking with people in a systematic fashion is one way to learn about the personal and social aspects of meaning and action that are blended into identity.

Identity is a combination of idiosyncratic (unique) and socially shared (common) meanings acquired, used, and applied to self and others during the continuous socialization that is a mainstay of human aging. One outcome of this interplay is the creation of a social location for identity and for the person—a social location that has the potential for being altered over the course of life. The distinguishing feature of identity is this recognizable location formed through a blending of personal and social meanings that tell the individual, I am here, I am this, I am that, at the same time they imply I am not there, I am not this, I am not that. Identity is much more than the combination of existential and intellectual knowledge of who I am; it is a boundary that marks where the person is found and where others begin. In modern societies, identity, across a lifetime, is not a permanently fixed or immutable location. In late life, as in earlier stages of childhood and adulthood, meaning is woven continuously into identity through symbolic interaction. Ideational domains such as those of religion, spirituality, or faith and the folkways and norms within those social worlds provide the abstract or theoretical framework for social life of individual and society.

Meaning plays a pivotal part in establishing the specific configuration and dynamic of identity. The interpretive process seated within the individual social actor is the key to creating and embracing a specific identity, especially in a modern (highly differentiated) society. Discerning the meaning and value of religious belief and behavior in late life rests on the epistemological assumption that the creation and use of meaning is an intrinsic part of social behavior and one that is indicated to the person and the listener during the interview. The objective in uncovering meaning is to understand not so much why people adopt religion, but how and in what ways and on what occasions religion enters into their lives. The way in which people define religion and learn about it is, of course, dependent upon the meanings they have internalized from a lifelong participation in culture and in myriad groups. In the blunt vernacular of the early 21st century, this study discerns and describes some of the ways that contemporary older adults "do" religion.

The discovery of how, when, and where religion is factored into daily life is brought to light in the conversation of the interview in yet another way. Strauss (1959, p. 145) has suggested that an active accounting of life is a crucial part of personal identity. "Each person's life, as he writes or thinks about it, is a symbolic ordering of events. The sense that you make of your own life rests upon what concepts, what interpretations, you bring to bear upon the multitudinous and disorderly crowd of past acts. If your interpretations are convincing to yourself, if you trust your terminology, then there is some kind of continuous meaning assigned to your life as-a-whole."

Interviews are contexts that engender symbolic ordering and provide a method and vehicle for glimpsing the domains of social meaning and interpretation of meaning that are within individual identity. It is in this manner that identity emerges as an observable social location composed of biographic (personal) and situated (social) features of the person. In some respects, proponents of developmental perspectives are likely to find the symbolic interactionist perspective compatible with the broadly construed themes they have posited; in particular, that meaning and identity are associated with analytically distinct stages of life which are themselves linked to aging. Stage theorists contend—in diverse vocabularies and with disparate theoretical models—that in the process of aging there are substantive and incrementally ordered changes in the meaning of self and identity (Buhler, 1968; Erikson, 1963; Gould, 1978; Levinson, 1978; Vaillant, 1977). Changes in age and in relationships necessitate changes in the kinds of psychic work to be completed in each stage of life. Hence, identities change as a function of the periodic taking up and completion of tasks that appear at various points along the life course.

Stage theories offer an important corrective to the idea of intrapsychic and interpersonal stagnation during younger years or ages. And some, like Erikson's model, laid a foundation for treating old age as a stage where development and identity culminated. The notable motif is that of old age as the last testing ground for the meanings given to the elder's own identity and the identities of others. Ego integrity, the positive resolution of late life's developmental work, "is the ego's accrued assurance of its proclivity for order and meaning. It is a post-narcissistic love of the human ego—not of the self—as an experience which conveys some world order and spiritual sense, no matter how dearly paid for . . . the possessor of integrity is ready to defend the dignity of his own life style against all physical and economic threats. In such final consolidation, death loses its sting" (Erikson, 1963, p. 268). Ego integrity is synonymous with a biographic and situated identity that is neither self-absorbed nor vicariously absorbed in others. All of this implies that old age is the stage of life where identity achieves an equilibrium that is genuinely human and humane and may be the prelude to Joan Erikson's ninth stage of gero-transcendence.

Although ego integrity is not a central feature of works accentuating the social aspects of individual identity, such an idea is not wholly alien to sociological study, if it is reconceptualized in terms involving character and social structure or in terms of mapping the individual's social location within social worlds and the interaction within those social worlds. For sociologists, part of this mapping of identity is closely related to the cohort or generational experience that shapes the structural possibilities for individuals. Van Gennep (1960), Mannheim (1952), Ryder (1965), Riley (1968, 1972), and Elder (1974) are a few of those whose work established a framework for this perspective.

Though it is possible to be shortsighted by adhering firmly to a structural model that posits an overly deterministic view of the power social forces wield in shaping human behavior (Wrong, 1961), it is necessary to consider their role in shaping generational, cohort, and personal experiences of individuals. Even the most coercive and inhospitable social structures and social contexts, ones seemingly impenetrable and unaffected by individual action, may be defined by individuals and understood as if they were movable, permeable, and subject to change. For example, in *Man's Search for Meaning*, Frankl (1963) states that the oppressive and unalterable reality of concentration camps did not release prisoners from the personal responsibility to make sense of their lives and the ghastly and unjust deaths they witnessed. Taking a stand (self-indication in the language of symbolic interaction) towards the meaning of these daily events in which they participated as victims— unwilling and coerced—was a vital way to retain a shred of personal and human identity. Those who did not have this "will to meaning" resigned themselves to the depersonalized and stunted identities forced upon them by others. Experiences in the death camps offer authentic if extreme examples of how the definitions individuals formulate about situations direct them to pay heed to one or more features of self and social setting, thereby shaping identity and life. It is logically possible, and perhaps ultimately necessary in late life, to create and live one's own identity rather than to adopt the identity proffered by others or by institutions. An enduring faith or religious involvement that lasts a lifetime may offer individuals a reserve source for invoking Frankl's will to meaning.

Age Homogamy and Identity

The experience of age homogamy (pursuing activities with spouses, colleagues, and neighbors who are close to one's own age as person and others move through the life course) in a society based on age norms and folkways, means that with the exception of health problems, and quitting full-time participation in the labor force, one may continue to relate to life as if surrounded by the collective experience of an earlier and an evolving generation or cohort (Mannheim, 1952). Elders observe that they and their friends are growing old together. Life changes, but a cohort or generational chunk of life also endures. This means that elders may be assured that they are not too much different from what they were at twenty or forty-five when they arrive at sixty-five, seventy-four, or ninety-two, particularly if there is someone close to them (and this someone might well be a sense of a connection to the divine) who sees and acts as if ostensibly submerged features of social and personal identity continue to be significant. Religion and faith duplicate or parallel societal patterns of interaction based on age. Hence, religion is conducive to supporting a kind of inertial guidance system among the old that reinforces the basic stability or continuity underlying personal and cohort ties to religious organizations and practices.

BIOGRAPHIC AND SITUATED ASPECTS OF FAITH IN LATE LIFE

To think expansively about identity is to build on the general premise mentioned previously, that identity is social location. Religious beliefs and behaviors, items James subsumed theoretically under the spiritual dimension of the self, are important dimensions across life and in terms of social and personal identity. Some contemporary psychodynamic perspectives on religion concur (Rizzuto, 1993). Research and publication on the relationship between religion and health among community elders (Idler, 1994) and the link with mental health examined by a number of researchers and research teams and principally identified with Koenig (1998) offer further support for the idea that religion, once decried as something that "seriously sabotages mental health" (Ellis, 1985, p. 5), has become a focus for ongoing study by scientists who once scoffed and scorned. Many of those efforts are based on survey research and other large-scale quantitative studies. Whereas some quantitative studies require face-to-face interaction with respondents, qualitative work features it as an intrinsic part of the research process. Thus, once the reasons for the study and the questions have been identified, the project moves inexorably to the field.

A METHODOLOGICAL LENS: PEOPLE IN THEIR NATURAL SURROUNDINGS

As one person said when greeting me at the door to her home, "I'm happy you found me. It's hard to find the house." This particular house was harder to find than most others; it was nearly invisible from a spot in a field where the street number was clearly posted. Reaching the house involved following a circuitous loop and a counterintuitive course to reach the other side of the field. This example is a graphic reminder that finding people in the field is literally and figuratively a step not nearly as straightforward as it initially appears to be. Yet finding people in their homes and obtaining some sense about the material and nonmaterial social surroundings that shape their daily life is an essential part of understanding the distinctive features faith has for each person; it provides the interviewer with a deeper appreciation for the places where people's lives unfold every day, and offers firsthand contact with the social and economic circumstances that fix the range of social interaction for daily life.

Qualitative research involves listening for, gathering, and giving voice to individual and group experience. Qualitative work ultimately transposes the unique notation of lives into a composition reflective of themes that characterize the group as a whole. The observations of behavior or the statements from individual interviews are integral parts of the analysis for the research but do not wholly constitute the unit of that analysis. This idea is expressed cogently in the words of a psychologist who once described her own work in collecting interviews, "as weak on statistics . . . but good at listening to human stories" (Gavron, 2000, p. 167).

Others like Liebow (1993) and Myerhoff (1980) have rendered definitive ethnographies about rich and complex relationships, that were obtained through processes of listening and interviewing as well as from participant observation. The observations and interviews of urban, homeless women, and Jewish elders, respectively, are exemplars for understanding the procedures and methodical steps involved in capturing stories of distinctive groups, groups often disregarded by those using other methodological approaches to the study of lives in those social worlds. Notwithstanding their insights, the focus of my research was a bit different from theirs in substance and in kind. The more elusive subject in this research project was an ordinary or typical older adult living in the community.

In a primer and compendium on feminist methods of social research (Reinharz, 1992, p. 50), the author quotes a passage from Helen Merrell Lynd's discussion of research progress in the classic community study, Middletown. Helen Lynd credits her co-researcher, Faith Williams, with moving the Middletown study from "generalities" to the rich and specific accounts of people's lives that were gathered and woven into the picture of life in an American community. Williams insisted that the research team talk directly with people in addition to detailing the behaviors researchers were observing and categorizing. Similar insights about the experiential and interactional features of the interview are also found in the phenomenological perspective articulated by Schutz (1970).

This idea of appreciating the "vocal nature of communication" has long been deemed important to those investigating the relationship between the individual and others. In his classic formulation of the clinical or psychiatric interview, Harry Stack Sullivan noted that clinicians would be well served by being "alert" to aspects of vocal communication, particularly " . . . signs or indicators of meaning . . . " that illuminated broader "patterns of living" (Sullivan, 1954, p. 5). As the composer and conductor Aaron Copland once noted with respect to the role of listening in music: "In a sense, the ideal listener is both inside and outside the music at the same moment, judging it and enjoying it, wishing it would go one way and watching it go another" (Copland, 1985, p. 19). The experiential dimensions surrounding the interview process are strongly linked to active listening, including aspects of vocal communication that trigger the words and perspectives disclosed in the exchange that occurs between an interviewer and an interviewee. Perhaps this is one reason to view qualitative work as a research process that uses a series of experiential filters as a way of understanding interaction and builds those filters into the process of studying social reality and transposing it into analysis and text. In participant observation, to some degree "the researcher becomes an instrument or the instrument of the research" (Liebow, 1993, p. vii). In some measure, the capacity to see with a third eye and to listen with a third ear are essential requirements for these approaches.

SELECTING PEOPLE FOR INTERVIEWS

Such heightened sensitivity to the qualitative process does not obviate the need to select older people for the study, especially those willing to tell the story of faith in their lives. The people interviewed in the study constitute what is ordinarily known in social science as a purposive or theoretical sample. Quite often it is also termed, a sample of convenience, though in my way of thinking that phrase is reserved for the perennial research projects that use college students, generally sophomores, as their sample. Notwithstanding the accuracy of all these terms as descriptors of this study, I also call this study and the selection process that guided it, a network sample, or one in which older people were approached about their willingness to participate in an interview through other nominees. That is, I asked a varied and sundry group of people to nominate or refer me to older adults who were likely to be receptive and open to talking about their family backgrounds and their experiences with religion. In addition, as I solicited names of prospective participants from this social network, I kept an eye on a few social characteristics that are relevant to social gerontologists, namely, sex, age, and residential status. There was also a deliberate attempt on my part to include nonwhite elders among those to be approached for an interview, just as there was an attempt to ensure that both economically privileged and less economically privileged elders were included in the study. In the main, the sample is one that evolved in the process of asking for names of men and women, aged sixty or older, living in the community who might be willing to meet with me to talk about religion and late life.

Although network nominations accounted for the majority of leads for interviews and resulted in the majority of actual interviews, there were a few internal snowball recommendations drawn from interviewees in the study. In one of the closing questions of the interview, each person interviewed was asked if he or she could refer me to someone else who might be willing to be interviewed. Four participants were nominated and interviewed via this snowball technique.

Tapping into this real-life social network anchored by the researcher was advantageous in that people were recommended by nominators who were themselves a fairly diverse group in terms of social roles and statuses. The outcome was that in a small sample there is a sufficient degree of variability among the people interviewed. Another advantage in using this anchored network to elicit nominees was that researcher credibility was vouched for by nominators and was built into the research process for all of the participants in the study, community or long-term care. This was important because I was not a member or insider in any of the social worlds studied; I was an outsider and a stranger to older adults I wished to interview. Nominators could allay any anxiety people might have about talking with a university professor who wanted to ask questions about old age and religion.

Exercising this network of relationships and contacts that existed among the nominators, the nominees, and the researcher, also enhanced the likelihood of developing rapport with those participating in the interviews. Most of us are reassured of the purpose and intent surrounding interaction when a neutral but credible person who has some link to ourselves and a third, unknown party or person, attests to what can be expected in a situation where we and someone not known to us will have a fairly long and intimate conversation. Older people who were nominated via this process welcomed the interviewer into the natural setting of their homes and living rooms. From the researcher's perspective, asking for recommendations from a wide variety of nominators in a super-network composed of smaller integrated networks (social, professional, community, and educational) provided a prescreening of the interviewee's credibility and capacity to respond to questions. Finally, the network of nominators was also a soundly vetted group in the sense that members had been known and trusted in their various social roles over many years by both the researcher and the older adult.

How Long-Term Care Institutions and Participants Were Selected

Finding people in long-term care facilities who were willing to talk about their lives and faith was both similar to and different from the method described above. Likely participants for interviews were nested, if you will, within long-term care facilities. Consequently, institutions with a willingness to entertain social research had to be identified and then approached about participation before participants were contacted. Six unique institutional facilities were part of the study. Four of the five facilities were settings for multiple interviews with people who received different levels of health care or assistance within the facility. One facility was the location for a single interview, while the sixth was exclusively a site for participant observation. I was familiar with two of the six facilities from years of contact and membership in a local group of gerontological practitioners and academic professionals. Three of the remaining four institutions were suggested by others as being open to research. The fourth institution was one I had no knowledge about prior to the study. There were repeated visits to four of the six sites, including the two facilities where separate observational work supplemented the interviews. In one of the two sites where observation occurred, I spent half a day in participant observation with a pastoral care person and had informal conversations with residents, but no formal interviews were held. Please see Appendix A for more detailed discussion of other ways in which the selection procedure varied from the procedure used among community-dwelling older adults.

By the end of the selection process, at the close of the study, interviews with 46 older adults, 31 from the community and 15 from long-term care facilities, had been completed and formed the base of the qualitative fieldwork for this book. In addition to interviews with the elderly, six formal observations of group interaction were completed and seven interviews with people connected to spiritual and religious programs for the elderly were conducted. All of the research work or fieldwork was completed in a year—August 24, 1999 to August 25, 2000. There were interviews with 31 women and 15 men. About 13% of the group or 6 people were nonwhites. Please see Appendix B for other information about specific characteristics of the sample.

The purpose of this qualitative study was to understand the kinds of religious beliefs and behaviors that were meaningful and salient to older adults within two residential settings (selected questions from the interview guide appear in Appendix A). Members of the sample or participants in the study were drawn to approximate in a microcosm the range of social characteristics among older adults in the state. The strength of this selection process or the positive feature of any bias in the selection is that people were comfortable about expressing their thoughts about faith and religion. They were from a welter of social backgrounds and resided now in very different social worlds, but a shared aspect of life as elders was found in their willingness to talk about the meaning and value of faith. They also shared three other important characteristics.

SHARED EXPERIENCES IN THE GROUP

Residential Longevity

As a way to highlight some of the factors and themes that emerged from the study, there are three items worth noting before the substantive discussion of the chapters that follow. One important feature is the enormous longevity older adults had in the state of Connecticut. When taking the larger region (New England, New York, New Jersey, Pennsylvania) into account, nearly everyone had moved to Connecticut a "lifetime" ago. There were a handful of people who had been born in other countries or in U.S. territories and another handful that had been born outside the state of Connecticut, but in the U.S. However, despite this variation in place of birth, nearly all had been residents of the state, and in many cases, their current communities for all or most of their lives.

Generational Status

When I started this research, as I met older adults and talked with them about religion and faith, I asked people if they thought of themselves as religious. Just as many who answered yes, answered no, and a few said they once were religious but now they could no longer could say that religion was meaningful to them. Interestingly enough, no one in this study "got religion" in the sense that they were irreligious or unchurched as children and young adults and then became religious or faithful in late life. With one or two exceptions, the older adults in the study were not seeking religion or hoping to find a new religious faith. For the most part, religion was given, taught, and accepted. Adjustments were added as necessary and incrementally. Religion was declined or rejected by only a few. This pattern is in stark contrast to the impulse and propensity documented by others of the journeys and quests that characterize Boomer cohorts.

Religions or faiths offer both the instrumental and expressive anchors of meaning for many among the current cohorts of older adults in the United States. For the majority of older adults, particularly those born before 1941, the beginning of direct U.S. involvement in World War II, the direct participation in mainstream religious organizations during childhood and young adulthood assured a connection to something larger than themselves. Present cohorts of the old are distinctive in their pattern of early childhood and continuing adult participation in faith and religion.

One of the most compelling points of Putnam's (2000) encyclopedic analysis of trends in voluntary participation among U.S. adults during the past century is that older adults are aging out in religious denominations and organizations, as is the case with other civic groups. Older participants and members are not being replaced by younger adults in an array of voluntary associations. As many have predicted, the now middle-aged, Boomer cohorts (1946–1964) have substantively different patterns of religious involvement and in the salience of their faith than do their elders. Current cohorts of older adults received direct socialization into the institutional and relational social worlds of religions and faiths during their childhood and early adulthood. Though the choice to remain outside those religious social worlds was present as a possibility from late young adulthood, and many in this generation moved through adulthood with periodically attenuated ties, the generation studied here differs in patterns of religiosity from those found in research on Boomer cohorts (Roof, 1993, 1999). Thus, the research goal of tapping into the reality of religious belief and behavior among older adults in typical community settings results in learning more about what older adults put into and take away from the practice of faith.

OLD AGE AS A TIME FOR LIVING

Despite this steadfast engagement with faith, the older adults in the study did not see themselves as religious paragons nor as unduly or auspiciously enlightened. The lines from Psalm 139, "See if my way is crooked and lead me in the way of old," capture the essence of the sample's perspective on God and the religious institutions that renew and transmit the ways of walking this path without going "crooked." The women and men in the study come from many denominational backgrounds from three major religions, or churches in the vocabulary of sociology or religion, Catholicism, Judaism, and Protestantism, that have shaped our society. They see themselves as people who have lived their lives in the hope of doing right by others and by themselves.

Though it is fashionable and flattering in some circles to see those who were young adults during World War II as exemplifying the "greatest" generation, no one here thought of themselves or described peers as constituting a superior generation, the best one, in terms of contemporary U.S. history. The youngest person interviewed was born in 1940, thus everyone interviewed had lived through the second world war, though several were mere infants, and others were children and adolescents during those years, and largely unaware of its impact on their daily lives. Instead of hubris, their words bespoke more modest attempts to live life in accordance with a sense of faith and by keeping in mind that there was a purpose to life—something beyond themselves, whether that something else was a divine force or a favorable disposition to the idea of duty and service and maybe even actually following through on service.

I see the people interviewed as being, in a phrase peppered throughout the Book of Psalms, as the "upright of heart," not so much because they deeply understood or even accepted religious and theological beliefs without question but because they expected to be engaged in faith as a part of life, and for the most part, they still are engaged in keeping some aspects of faith alive and vital. The involvement with religion is not ecstatic or ephemeral nor is it vague or mysterious. They are connected to religious belief and behavior across the life course through enduring and meaningful social interactions and layers of it perhaps more than they are tethered by a transcendent link alone. They can see that younger generations are not as firmly linked to folkways of faith, and this seems regrettable to them but not a hallmark of failure that can be attributed to them, or for that matter to the young.

Many people in this study commented that "with God you are never alone." Though not everyone intends to personalize God with this statement, and many older adults do not hold a personalized image of God, it is the referential link to the idea of the sacred across life that endures even at the end of life. Interestingly, for those who call themselves atheists or agnostics, the idea of the sacred had been supplanted by other non-deistic but equally powerful and perhaps transcendent links. This goes a long way toward understanding that death is not generally a topic that preoccupies older adults in the sample.

In writing this book, I've frequently been asked, What do people say about death? Well, they actually said little about death. Some had a great deal to say about the technology and prolongation of death, and others were concerned about pain and suffering. There was also animated discussion of recent funerals of people who were friends and relatives, and sadness acknowledged in talking about losses over the years of people and animals who were special and significant to the person. But the talk of death itself was realistic and down-to-earth. There was not the fuss and bother about death that many presume is a universal feature of late life. Instead, the outlook of older adults in this study resonates in these lines from "Courage" by the poet Anne Sexton (1975, p. 16).

> when death opens the back door
> you'll put on your carpet slippers
> and stride out.

Readers have now crossed the front doors and thresholds into the homes and rooms of the older adults in the study. It is time to stride into an extended discussion of what people said about their lives and the folkways of faith that enfold them.

CHAPTER TWO

The Bedrock of Faith and Religion—Socialization

"It's like a habit."

Religious affiliation is part of the social legacy created for individuals through marriage and the unique composition of the family of origin. Religious affiliation and the biographical bedrock of an individual's religious identity is shaped through the active work of a wider network of kin, biological or social, who provide face-to-face interaction over the course of childhood and adolescence to children and young adults in their charge and in their care. Nearly every older adult in the study was raised in a nuclear family setting, biologically based and socially legitimated, but a few grew up in family-like settings with guardians who provided socialization to religion. One's initial religious affiliation is ascribed or given at birth. Over the course of a person's life religious affiliation may be changed. Thus, religious statuses and roles are both ascribed (bequeathed at birth) and achieved (chosen or selected by the individual).

In this study there was ample evidence in recollections about parents and family, as well as in a person's description of what life was like during childhood and early adulthood, that official religious affiliation had changed for many over the course of their lives. But the changes described were not dramatic switches to religions found at the extreme ends a religious continuum, for instance, moving from Baptist to Shinto, nor were they cavalier responses to disaffection with one's ascribed religion. It is also worth mentioning that no one in this group of elders was unchurched or without systematic exposure to religious experience during childhood or youth, and that for this group, switching religious affiliation meant joining another religious group rather than moving into apostasy. Moreover, most switching occurred for specific reasons and involved moving relatively small distances within the realm of Christian denominations. This does not mean that people had similar depth and comprehensive exposure to religious beliefs and behaviors during childhood or adulthood, nor does it mean that their religious upbringing was viewed in uniformly flattering or unflattering terms. It does mean that everyone interviewed had exposure to and experience with religion and religious social worlds over a fair number of years at the outset of their lives.

This kind of socialization is what I call bedrock socialization. It was a pervasive, and as the elders say in their own words, inescapable, feature of growing up. The depth of this religious bedrock is important to consider in terms of another key characteristic of the group interviewed, the longevity of residence in the state of Connecticut and often in their residential communities or hometowns. In other words, one of the special features of the group, noted in chapter 1, is the fact that many were born, were raised, and lived most if not all of their lives within the New England region or more typically in the state of Connecticut.

There were people who had immigrated from outside the U.S.; some had immigrated as young people and others as adults. Others had moved to the state from other states many years ago. There was also a person who spends a good portion of the year in Connecticut with younger family members and the rest of the year in a U.S. territory. Less than a handful maintained part-time residences in warmer climes within the U.S. This feature of the sample, longevity of residence, is a sociological key to understanding the many ways that elders kept connected to faith (again, sometimes not the same faith of childhood, but a slightly different one) over the course of their lives. Among the oldest members of this study, active involvement and connection with the faith of their childhood was approaching the century mark. It is a clear but still compelling feature of the objective situation of people's lives when religion and faith have been part of those lives across a century of massive social changes and attendant turning points of human history.

The robust quality of these beliefs and behaviors is something to be reckoned with even if it is difficult to capture in well-defined bits of measured units. In other words, were these same interview questions to be posed to their elderly counterparts in different areas of the country with significantly shorter residential histories and greater rates of immigration, the concept of bedrock socialization, and consistent involvement with religion might not emerge. During the early 19th century Connecticut acquired the appellation of "the land of steady habits" (Mathews, 1951, p. 954). One of the steadiest habits in this group of contemporary older adults is that of religious affiliation and participation, for though some within this generation have moved away from faith, most have continued in practices built on the bedrock of socialization in childhood and young adulthood.

Indeed, Ed's description of his involvement with religion from childhood until the present, "It's like a habit," doesn't convey the simultaneous wonder and wry tone of his voice when he made this statement. Religiosity, for people in this study, is not a quality to herald as worthy of admiration or as a way of setting themselves apart for special consideration. It is a hallmark of belonging and of finding over the course of life that their understandings and even their ways of "doing" faith might change, but that the beliefs and behaviors absorbed into self and identity long ago remained important in terms of participation and in principle. There is a comprehensiveness to the religious belief and behavior they describe and detail in their retrospective and contemporary accounts about involvement with religion.

From the retrospective accounts about childhood and young adulthood much is learned about the mostly continuous but occasionally revised aspects of a person's understanding and practice of religion. A picture emerges of the value assigned to faith in daily life and to the content of that life. A biographical, generational baseline is established that gives the person, the interviewer, and now the reader a sense of salience and stability attached to folkways of faith. The beginnings of this bedrock socialization occurred early in the last century during a time when greater numbers of Americans shared their daily lives within the context of community. The key features of early socialization to religion are the next items of discussion.

WORDS AS A FIRST LESSON IN FAITH

Regardless of specific religious affiliation, Catholic, Jew, or Protestant, people recall learning prayers from their mothers. Virtually all credited their mothers as the first person to teach them prayers and the first to guide them into saying their prayers daily, or in some cases, with teaching the formal religious prayers said regularly but not daily in the home. Though two people mentioned that grace (a prayer offered before meals) was said before each family meal, grace was not described as a regular form of prayer practiced in their childhood homes. Like Douglas, many came from large families where a host of other things were of immediate concern. "No, we didn't have time. When you've got to eat with nine, ten people sitting at a table, the food would come and you'd grab. My father would eat first, my mother always last. My mother was always serving. I never saw my mother sitting down to eat."

The prayers mothers taught were standard prayers central to Christian religions, and in some cases, to specific Jewish traditions. Mothers were also the supervisors of daily prayer, overseeing its practice. They were the line coaches for prayers taught in formal religious settings, such as special prayers associated with sacred turning points like Confession, Communion, and Confirmation. In this generation, all born before World War II, prayers were the first vocabularies and forms learned for talking with God. Mothers inculcated the words and sentences that children learned as special ways to ask for blessings upon family and friends, for expressing thanks, and for asking questions. Though a few elders no longer pray in the ways taught to them as children and young adults, prayer itself was and is the most common way of practicing faith for these older adults. In this study, prayer emerged as a significant dimension of religion in late life. Much more will be said about prayer in late life in chapter 4. We now turn to childhood in order to trace the initial process of socialization to religion. People had various appraisals of the experiences that befell them in the process of learning religious beliefs and behaviors, but nearly everyone remembered the experiences in depth and detail—right down, in many cases, to the generally beloved, and less frequently, excoriated, Sunday school teacher.

THE USUAL CAST OF SIGNIFICANT OTHERS AND THEIR ROLES IN THE PROCESS

MOTHERS MOST OF ALL, FATHERS RARELY, AND TEACHERS FOLLOWING BOTH

Inasmuch as mothers were credited as primary teachers, fathers were not spoken of as significant others or role models for religious socialization. No one spoke, for example, of fatherly instruction in prayer or of a direct role that fathers played in overseeing religious development. This may very well speak to the more rigidly defined sex roles that prevailed in the family culture and larger society surrounding older adults when they were children and young adults. Even so, there were one or two notable exceptions to this pattern.

Edward, 60, the youngest member of the study, recalled that "every Sunday just like clockwork" the family's day was shaped by mass. His mother went to mass early in order to prepare Sunday dinner; later his father went to church, "in a suit," for the 11 o'clock mass. His father would stop at the railroad station to have his shoes polished every Sunday before going to church. Edward recalls his curiosity as a child about the miracles conveyed by the nuns in their religious education classes. He sees religion then and now as "Something that had to be done, and I did it, and I still do it. It's like a habit." Anne's father also played a central role in her socialization. "Well actually, I think that my parents, when we were young, always felt prayer was important. They were not overbearingly strict, although my father, we always went to mass, which was mostly with my father. My mother would go several times a year, okay, Christmas, Easter. However, she, in her way, had a very, she was very involved with prayer in her own way. What happened? She had a very sad experience with a priest in Italy that kind of threw her for a loop, let's just say. She never got quite back on track. And she felt uncomfortable after that going to mass because of that one experience." Here the father became the active teacher, a role unusual among the accounts that older adults told regarding their early religious experiences.

Sally, a first generation American who is Roman Catholic, recalls attending "mass every Sunday. And when it was May and October, May Devotion—if we were outdoors playing baseball when that church bell rang, you dropped everything, and you ran home, ran in with dirt on your face, and you went to church, or you had an explanation." Sally's mother taught the prayers in Polish. Her mother was the keeper of all religious traditions, "I don't think it was my father. It was all my mother." Wanda learned prayers at home and recalls formal religious instruction this way, "We had the catechism, and with the Catholic religion, what I don't like about that is that they teach us catechism. You just memorize everything but you don't understand much, you know. I bet half of us didn't know what was going on. But with the Protestants, they work more on the Bible, which is better, I think."

Some men in the study had filled special religious roles during childhood. This was true of Patrick, a Roman Catholic. He describes serving as an altar boy for most of his youth. "I always made, I always made mass. I always served it and made it, if I didn't, my sister and I went [attended without serving]. When I got older and we had mass every day at noon, well, I used to go to mass every day during Lent." When asked what was the best thing about being an altar boy, he answered, "Well it was just, that you felt your religion, [you were] a little closer to your religion than you would be otherwise." In his case the early experience of "being closer" meant that during World War II, when he was in his thirties, he voluntarily took on the role of assisting the hard-pressed chaplains. Thus, the socialization and special role played in youth had both durability and meaning across his life. Today it is precisely this contact and celebration as part of a closely-knit group that he misses and longs to find somehow in the long-term care facility where he lives.

There were many elders like Patrick who had been active in taking on formal roles within their faith and congregation even as young people. Barbara, for example, was also a joiner and participant. "I was quite active in the church in the nursery and I went to the graves, and we were confirmed about 12 and had our first communion. I belonged to the Girls' Friendly, the [youth group]. I was a joiner. Yes, and some of those people are still my friends today. . . . We always get together at least once a year, usually in July. . . . There used to be about thirty but it's down to about ten." For many older adults, active religious roles filled since childhood and ones they continued to fill as they aged are often unavailable to them in late life, particularly if their residence is now a nursing home.

Another account, this from Rose, 68, highlights the role of significant others in religious socialization during childhood and evokes the ways in which religion was woven into the daily and seasonal social life of family and community. After the death of her mother and her grandparents, a Roman Catholic godmother "was the one who used to take me to church." This was the one positive relationship Rose had as a child with an adult. Rose did sewing and seamstress work at home with an aunt. They made gloves and nightgowns and the pay they received was "very bad." Through the translator Rose says that "she used to pray to the Virgin Mary and God and [in this way] she felt her mother was watching her. And that's what kept her away from doing things that she would have done, could have done. Her mother from heaven [protected her]." Rose tells the translator that those beliefs and ideas were "a nice kind of ignorance, that helped her survive." The saints' festivals are especially memorable for her as celebrations and joyous events, because she does not otherwise have "happy memories of childhood." This feature of religion as a separate world or institution woven so tightly into the fabric of community life that community and religious involvement were almost fused, was one noted by others as a dominant characteristic of their childhood and young adult experience with faith. As Rose observes, the tight weave of religion and community once combined to offer experiences that added something special to the life of participants, something separate but closely connected to family that was, in some cases, even better than the experiences their families were able to provide.

Rose and Sally as well as several others learned their first prayers and religious lessons in a language other than English. Sometimes these first lessons were in the U.S. and sometimes in their native land. For example, Eugene, whose first language was Gaelic, came from a family of twelve in a rural area of Ireland where his elementary schooling occurred in a three-room schoolhouse. This was followed by formal instruction in a Christian Brothers school until he finished school at 17. He and a sister left Ireland in 1947 because "we needed a better way of living." His mother is credited as the person who had the most influence on his religious socialization. "She taught us wrong from right. She taught us how to pray and how to be religious." He understands Gaelic and can speak it, but has only occasional opportunities to put the language to use nowadays.

The ethnic background among the elders varied in a way that is consistent with their generational status and the representation of ethnic groups in the southern New England region. Spanish, Portuguese, Slavic, Russian, Gaelic, German, Italian, French, some Scandinavian languages, and Yiddish were primary languages in the home and were part of many childhood socialization experiences, including religious ones. Although the use of these languages in the home was a central feature of childhood, it was one that predictably was lost, except in rare instances, as people grew older. One person who learned prayers at home in French from her mother was surprised to admit, "I forgot the French. Funny, I forgot them in French though. I'd have to review them in French. I know the Hail Mary. Yes, I know that one. But I don't know the Father; I forgot it. But I used to know all of those. The Cradle, I knew all of those in French. I'd have to review it. It would take me about five minutes to review it. I'd catch it though I'd get it right back." Despite her optimism about recapturing fluency, only a few elders continued to use a language other than English for prayer, and this was in a very limited fashion for a small repertoire of prayers. A few Roman Catholics regretted the loss of mass in their familial language, for instance, Polish or Portuguese, but only two registered any regret about the loss of the Latin mass. Finding such a strong adaptation to institutional changes in religious ritual was mildly unexpected, simply because Latin and non-English services had been regular features of formal participation in religious worship for many Roman Catholics during much of their childhood and adulthood.

Others, such as Douglas, report some mixed messages from childhood religious socialization. Yes, it provided a stability which they recognize as having been largely beneficial to them, but often the lessons, religious and secular, were not given in an affectionate way. "Oh, we were brought up very strict. . . . The school, the nuns at school were unbelievably strict. They, at six, seven, eight years old, they'd take you by hand on first Friday of the month, take you to confession. What does a six, seven-year-old got to confess about? You know, they drummed it in to you. Didn't hurt. It didn't hurt, but it really left a label on, it left a message. Oh no, they were very strict. And during Lent, I remember even now at home, during Lent, every night after supper my father and mother would kneel down. And we'd all kneel on a hardwood floor, whatever floor we were on and say the rosary. . . . Oh yes. And my father would get the Bible and read it to himself and once in a while he'd tell—give us a passage of what he read. He would try to analyze it or see what you thought of it or, . . . he'd give his view of it."

The more prevalent perception and account of fathers and their role in religious socialization is found in seventy-five-year-old Julia's emphatic statement: "My father: the only time he ever went to church was weddings and funerals and christenings." Her mother was the religious influence for Julia, who was raised Methodist, although her parents originally were Episcopalian or Presbyterian. Her religious exposure was broadened when she attended and graduated from a Roman Catholic secondary school for girls. She later finished her baccalaureate and a master's degree on the same campus many years later when it had become a private college. As she says, "and it's funny, I've never become a Catholic. But yet think of the influence the Catholic church has had on my life." Taking it one notch further than Julia, in terms of her father's presence in religious socialization, Ellen says: "I don't think my father was in a church after he got married, but mother did. And mother had a strong faith." Beth put it even more succinctly, "My father always said he was good. He didn't have to go to church."

A few spoke about a more subtle influence and role played by their fathers in this process of shaping religious identity. For instance, Margaret attributes her foundation of faith to her mother, but as we converse, it is clear that the father's support was important in the process, albeit indirectly. He was a firm supporter of Margaret's religious development as it was inculcated by her mother. "I think it was the way I was raised by a devout mother and a wonderful father, who was not Catholic (he was German Lutheran), but reared us as Roman Catholics—my sister and I. So, I think the basis there was the training they had given us. . . . He was very strict, as far as our attendance at church and Sunday School and everything." Others also mentioned a joint parental support for religion and schooling that was tempered by the disadvantages of social class, as did Alice who grew up "in a small mining town, not far from where they have the groundhog report. We moved to Connecticut when I was ten years old. I'm Catholic. Roman Catholic. My parents always had us go to a parochial school. I always went—as far as the ninth grade. The Depression—you had to go out and work—and I did housework at the age of fourteen." Another father felt the press of honoring the sacred and of taking care of his family. Sarah, 96, recalls her father's dilemma between supporting religion by attending the synagogue and his obligation to support his family. She describes religion as a serious part of her family, "Especially my mother. My father not so much. He used to think you're not supposed to work on Saturday. So, he'd get us up like he was going to services, and then he would change and he would go to work [he was a painter and paperer]. . . . But in the house he was strict."

The role of formal socialization and a wide-ranging and direct exposure to religions other than the one followed by the family played out in a different way for another member of the sample. Libby was the only child of a family with long roots in Millerville. This nineteenth century heritage might go unremarked in the larger community were it not for the fact that her religious roots were Jewish. One of the most highly educated members of the study, she had first graduated from a high school that was a private, religious academy. "You know, it's very funny. [laughs] We used to have chapel every morning . . . we'd march in and we'd have chapel. Of course, I was Jewish and this was an Episcopal school, in those days. Now, under the Episcopal Diocese, when we graduated, the bishop gave us our diplomas. Nevertheless, every morning a minister from either St. John's church or one of the Episcopal chapels would come in, and we would have—you know, we'd sing a hymn. Nobody made me sing. That was my choice, and I had a choice, anyway, but I learned all the hymns just the same. And they were lively. They were fun." She added, "You know, we had a reading from the Bible—either the Old Testament or the New Testament, with some kind of explanation that went with it. And I'd listen very carefully and learn a lot. . . . And I feel to this day, that it made me a more broad-minded person to do this."

Alex, also Jewish, and Libby's husband, described a childhood in Poland that was shaped if not wholly dominated in memory by the town's creation of a ghetto for Jews, where "really everybody lived from day to day." There was hunger and disease in the ghetto. "We had no place to pray. We prayed in the houses . . . you'd just pray in our house or your house, wherever there was room for ten people." Before 1939 there had been three synagogues in the town. However, the anti-Semitism steadily worsened and affected everyone when a group of Poles " . . . got some kind of an order . . . that said, "You can get yourself three hundred young Jews from the [town's] ghetto and put them to work on your property to dry your swamp. . . . So, they did it! They figure they got the big piece of land, they put some [drainage in]. . . . They got three hundred young Jews. And we used to fix it, trenches, big trenches, trenches, like this [arms outspread at shoulders about five to six feet]. And then we used to nail sticks every foot or two feet, and you'd go up and grab willows. And you used to weave [fencing]. . . . And one day, they eliminated the ghetto. . . . I wasn't there. My parents were there, and everybody else was." A sister "went over the fence and became an alien, like I did. But I was left in a camp over there. But we knew that it was just a question of time—that they would eliminate the camp."

Joan, who was born in Romania and later spent her childhood in Russia, also describes a cultural context that was inimical to the open practice of Judaism and permeated by anti-Semitism. "I had a tutor. Even the Jewish—I never went to the school, Hebrew School. Because they didn't allow any churches, or they didn't allow any synagogues. We didn't have a church or a synagogue. They closed them all down. Or they burned them down or they closed them down. But we went through—we had to hide in the cellars. We didn't have much to eat at that time, you know." Once family members had managed to leave Russia in successive waves, they eventually settled in Millerville. At that time, decades ago, the Jewish community in Millerville was thriving and Joan fondly remembers that once there was even a Jewish restaurant and several kosher butchers. Yet it is interesting to note that 96-year-old Ruth, who also grew up in Millerville's Jewish community, recalls that though she did not attend the Hebrew Institute, as her brothers had, she learned Hebrew even in an orthodox family. "There was a big synagogue on Kingsbury Street. That was a synagogue. They had a type of a balcony for the women and pillars. Orthodox. There was a Hebrew Institute next door. Now, I did not go to that Hebrew Institute [as her brothers had]. But my parents—I don't know where they scraped the money up, but they sent me to a private cheder, and the only other girl was Essie Rubin." The experience of anti-Semitism was inextricably bound up with memories of childhood for all of the Jewish elders who had immigrated to the U.S. As a child in Lithuania, 96-year-old Sarah said, "Well, I had a private teacher for Yiddish and then my mother tried to get me to the regular school and . . . somehow, she managed to get me in. But the kids made it so miserable. You know, 'Dirty Jew,' and all that kind of stuff. So, after a while, I quit . . . I was taught at home."

Others recalled a childhood where they were reminded at home and sometimes elsewhere that they were different from most others in terms of ethnicity and religion. In recounting her experiences, Carol, 79, reflects on both of these. "The family was close, really. And so, I was raised in a family where faith was very important. Because both my parents had come here from Ireland. And at the time, there were signs posted that there were jobs. And they would put, 'Irish need not apply.' So, they really faced an awful lot when they came here from another country. . . . And I guess that's what makes me—I'm calm and quiet. But oh, sometimes. You know, because you've got to stand up for yourself a little bit in this world, you know. You can't always turn the other cheek." As befits the complicated picture of intergroup relations in U.S. society, Sarah remembered that she was aware of hostility directed toward her because of her religion. In her case it was, "The kids . . . growing up in a mixed neighborhood. I was raised in a [predominantly] Jewish neighborhood. But across the street, there was an Irish family, and boy—those kids—the Irish kids—they hated the Jews." These experiences and the general awareness of "being different" in terms of the childhood-era's Protestant norm were significant enough to be recalled by a few, but as was the case with black elders, the experiences were not of the degree and magnitude to have carried over into identity in such a way that they had become the most telling feature of orienting oneself to others. It may also be that these keenly felt realities of childhood when religious and ethnic bigotry were more pervasive and socially acceptable in our society had been addressed or resolved in some ways by older adults. Among the black elderly in the study, experiences of discrimination and prejudice were noted more in terms of ethnicity or color than of religion. For some, the experiences of discrimination were mitigated by a lifelong engagement in exclusively black congregations that had also been active in bringing issues of racial equality forward as a part of their larger community and social activities.

Recollections of family participation in religious activities surrounding the major holidays of respective religions were warm in tone, although they were not particularly detailed or the focus of spontaneous or extensive remarks or observations. Roman Catholics recalled the month of May and evenings spent saying the rosary as a group to honor Mary. The preparations their mothers made for Passover were recounted by all of the Jewish women in the sample. Though parental and family involvement in faith set the standard for religious belief and behavior, it is important to note that during childhood the socialization experiences were not always uniform or without variation from what was typical. Libby, for one, "went to the Sunday school at the age of three [a grandmother taught Sunday school]. And stayed there until I was confirmed at the age of fifteen. No, not a Bat Mitzvah. The reformed did not have Bar and Bat Mitzvahs in those days. They do now." "My mother kept a kosher home because her parents wouldn't drink a cup of tea in the house if she didn't [keep kosher]." However, she adds, "But it was not an observant home because my father was brought up in a not observant home. But his mother never ate pork, never had any pork products in the house. So, everybody makes his own degree of observance. A very wise rabbi once said, 'Every Jew makes his own religion,' and that's really true." Libby talks about the fact that since her father bought Christmas toys to sell in his retail business their family always opened some presents on Christmas. "It had no religious significance. It was just a fun thing. And I did get Christmas presents. I got Chanukah presents from my mother's family—you know, grandfather and grandmother and maybe an aunt—and my father gave me Christmas presents. He used to bring home stuff from the store, all wrapped up in red paper. I opened it on Christmas morning. He brought it home on Christmas Eve and I opened it on Christmas morning. That's the best of all worlds."

One or two others had a similar, more broad exposure to religions than was true for most members of the study. As a child, Ellen recounts, she was raised in Christian Science. "My mother had gotten into it because she had come from Whitford, New York, which was a smaller town, of course, than Samuelson, and a very friendly town. . . . So she had gone to first one church and another to try to find one she thought would be a good one to, you know, but people were so cold. They weren't friendly and it hurt her. So a neighbor, and we eventually called her Auntie June, was in Christian Science. And so she got Mother interested. Mother never joined. We never joined it but we, that was primarily, that's where we went to Sunday school and if we were sick, well, we'd call a practitioner. But then my mother would say to the practitioner, 'Now you understand my husband insists that I get a doctor too.' And it [the church] was very popular, very busy. We would have standing room only at the second church. . . . I still use my lessons book from Christian Science. Even when I was travelling around I'd carry it with me, and read the lesson every, usually once a week."

TEACHERS RECALLED FROM 'SUNDAY' SCHOOL OR RELIGIOUS DAY SCHOOLS

Formal instruction from Sunday school teachers, Christian and Jewish, or from tutors, was mentioned as the second source of learning how to speak with God, after mothers and grandmothers. Teachers were the authoritative sources of explicit instruction about behavior in church and for formal religious rituals. It was somewhat surprising to me that several older adults remembered their Sunday school teachers clearly and offered rather detailed anecdotes about the kinds of formal and more often, informal, lessons they learned through religious education. One man had a special reason for clear recall. "My dad was a Sunday school teacher at [a local Protestant] church. [laughs] So I went to Sunday school there, naturally. And I had some good Sunday school teachers." He continued by naming several former teachers, and described the field trips that were part of his childhood religious instruction in the local congregation. Others also shared some lasting impressions of teachers and also of some of their classmates. This experience was recalled as an important part of childhood and one that was equally important among the older adults whose relatives had not been formal teachers of their faiths.

A handful of older adults had been centered in their religion to such an extent that as relatively young adults they became teachers and taught in the various denominations' Sunday schools. The former teachers had fond memories of those activities not merely for the sake of their students, but for what that experience brought to their understanding of religion and to practice of faith. Three people had taught religious education for some length of time at various stages of their lives, reflecting a high level of interest and commitment to passing on the traditions of faith to younger people.

As young people, only a few elders had close contact for extended periods of time with clergy from their religious communities. Though some elders had family members who were in fact, clergy, clergy members were not mentioned prominently as the source of religious education or as primary sources for learning to talk with God. With few exceptions, clergy formed an outer and distant set of social actors for socialization to faith among children and young people in the accounts provided by older adults. They did not figure prominently in the accounts older adults offered about key figures in learning about their faith or religion.

PARENTAL AND FAMILY CHANGES IN RELIGIOUS AFFILIATION

Some people recalled that their parents had switched religions. The word convenience may aptly describe some of the impetus for a change as long as it is recognized that availability of denominations may have been an equally important factor affecting religious choice and subsequent socialization. One example is given by Andrew, who has some reason to believe that his parents, both immigrants from England in the late 1800s, were originally Presbyterian. However, as he says, "we ended up Congregationalists. We had a Congregational chapel in Pequot Rapids." Today, he and his wife have been members for 66 years of a local Congregational church which, as Andrew phrases it, has changed "ownership" over the years as membership declined and two formerly distinct congregations merged into one. Aging in religious congregations is a kind of survivorship, as it is in other organizations. The bittersweet part of this longevity is that Andrew and his wife, Lydia, also interviewed in the study, have "outlived everyone who was once a member" of a service club that had been the social backbone of the congregation. They miss people who had been part of their lives. Lydia finds more meaning in formal worship, whereas Andrew says, "My feeling is a little bit more mild than hers, and mine is that going to church is as much being a part of the life of our friends as it could be. My feeling is that being with my friends at church is much more—means much more than if I were to go to another church. It's partly being with our friends—that is my view."

CHILDHOOD CHANGES OF FAITH: LOCATION, LOCATION, LOCATION

The theme of location was linked to safety for Walter and his choice of religious affiliation. His is a fascinating tale of choice because he did not know his biological parents and came to live with foster parents who were his guardians and defined his faith. "From the age of five, I went to Central Congregational Church in Riverside. I have a very funny reason why. Because the people I lived with were Episcopalians. But to go to the Episcopalian Church, I had to cross two major streets. Or, I could leave their house and walk up Middle Street without having to cross any major streets, to the center, and Middle Congregational Church. So, that's how I became a Congregationalist. And I have been all my life."

The various threads of religious identity and the dynamic nature of what it is all too tempting to view as a straightforward ascriptive process is evident in the biography of Phillip. His father was Methodist, his mother a Presbyterian. "And she was originally a Congregationalist here in town. And my, when [chuckles] my mother and dad were married, why, he gave in to her [laughs] I guess that's the way when you get married . . . so they went to the Congregational church at first. And my brother and my sister were baptized at the Congregational church, but he [the father] never felt at home there because he had been brought up at the Methodist church here in town. And so he finally convinced my mother that, 'Let's shift over to the Methodist church,' and so when I came along I was baptized with the Methodist church. [laughs] And then when, some years later, when my wife and I came up from [a large city] why she was a Congregationalist so we went to the Congregational church here."

EPIPHANIES

Though it was a unique experience in terms of the group as a whole, there was one person who described a change in her faith while she was young. As a girl, 90-year-old Clara started out in a Baptist church. "Then, when I was about twelve years old, there was an evangelist that came into the town and we all went to that. Well, I went there. My mother and I went. We went to the altar and got saved at the Pentecostal Church. My father didn't follow until quite a long time afterwards. Eventually, he did." The family went every Sunday to church and revivals, and Clara recalls that one "winter there were two hundred in the town that joined the church." This was long before radio or television were available. Indeed, she met her husband as a result of joining and participating in this new church.

Several people in the study had converted during childhood or young adulthood, moving from the ascriptive status provided by their parents or guardians to a religious affiliation they chose. Among those who actually converted, the achieved statuses or shifts were mostly between denominations within Protestantism that are relatively close to one another; a much smaller number moved across the Protestant and Roman Catholic divide. The latter movement occurred in both directions, although it is generally thought that the temper of the times was more supportive of movement from Protestant to Roman Catholic, particularly when marriage was involved. One childhood conversion is important to discuss because as an exception to the pattern of adult shifts in religious affiliation, it illustrates some important insights into points now being discussed about the formation of religious identity. Typically conversions were associated with the transition to marriage and family roles of early adulthood in order to raise children within one denomination. James's experience is an example of childhood conversion that is all the more interesting because it occurred within a family steeped in religion and in a family that actively shaped ways of thinking about religious values and service for many others. "Well, I, that's very interesting. My grandfather was a Methodist minister. In fact, he started the Samaritan Centers [a nationally and internationally recognized religious organization that emphasizes social outreach activities]. And he started the Samaritan [in Boston] and then he started the second Samaritan in Brooklyn. I worked there for a short time and my father was the executive director. They used to have a place in the Bowery, to take care of the drunks, you know that come in, and they'd work in the Samaritan for clothes and so on. And my grandmother did all the cooking for them. And we had as many as 200 men sleeping every night in Brooklyn. . . . They would come across the bridge from the Bowery [to work].

"When I was nine we had a family who lived across the street from us. I grew up with them and they were Catholic. And they would go to mass every Sunday, you know. And I got to know the one girl. The other girls went to Lady of Charity, a Catholic school. But this other one, she went to the public school like I did. We got to know each other and so on. So I, of course, the Catholics and the Protestants, a great divide at that time—tremendous. And I went to mass with her a couple times and I liked it. And I thought it offered me more, and yet I grew up in a Methodist church, and I went to Sunday school and I went to this and that. And I was only nine when I joined the Catholic church. I went through the [specific educational] program and my mother and father said, 'Whatever you want to do, it's up to you.' . . . Well, my father was, you know, he dealt with all kinds of people at the Samaritan and they were mostly people [needing help] obviously . . . and he met a lot of different people, you know, Jewish and Catholic and, you know, Lutheran and everything. And so he was fairly liberal in that sense. He was nonsectarian, really. He kept it that way, you know. And they had a chapel service every morning. People would go to chapel service every morning and some days it would be a priest. Some days they would have a rabbi. You know, some days they would have a Lutheran. He'd have all different, what's the word I'm looking for, religious, come and speak to his people in the morning." He goes on to relate that among friends who were boys, "They were all Methodists. You know, we grew up together. We went to Sunday school together. We went here; we went there. They all married a Catholic girl. In fact, I get letters from them all the time telling me jokes and things, you know. And, but wasn't that strange? There were five of us and they all married Catholic girls when they got married."

SWITCHING DENOMINATIONS AT MARRIAGE

More common than changing faith as a child, is the pattern of switching denomination at the point of marriage in young adulthood. Robert, 85, details his denominational shift as it is associated with marriage and the idea of forming a new family. His parents were German immigrants who spoke German at home. He called his mother, in a complimentary tone, the "Bible reading individual." His father was not as concerned with religion. Robert was raised as a "German Lutheran" and had lessons in German in preparation for his confirmation in 1928. When Robert married, he found that switching to his wife's Congregationalist denomination was not a giant leap, and he has been a very active member of his current congregation for 48 years. There also was a clear pattern in this study; that is, husbands shifted or converted to the denominational affiliation or congregation of the wife. Perhaps this was merely a form of emulation of the patriarchal behavior they experienced within their families, and this shift anticipated the reality in their own generation that women, this time their own wives, would continue to establish and set the standards for familial religious observance and the transmission of faith. Like the shifts in affiliation at other points in the life course, the shifts at marriage were proximate shifts among Christian or Jewish denominations. Gigantic leaps or apostasy were not described, nor do they characterize this group as a whole.

WHAT WAS GIVEN IS LATER RETURNED

Though there were not many elders in the sample who spoke of this, two older adults noted that in caring for their elderly parents they were careful to meet and attend to specific religious needs of their parents. These were spontaneous thoughts that occurred to them as they answered many of the questions about childhood and youth. Jean, for example, ensured that her elderly mother had opportunities to participate in religion when she cared for her mother [her mother lived with Jean and a sister until the mother's death in her late 80s]. This meant that Jean coordinated pastoral care and visits as well as television viewing of religious programs that her mother wished to see. They also said the rosary together, a practice her mother had followed throughout her life and one that her daughter had absorbed and now shared with her aged mother.

VARIATIONS IN DEPTH AND COMPREHENSIVENESS OF RELIGIOUS INVOLVEMENT

"RAISED IN THE CHURCH"

Six people were, as they called it, "raised in the church"; that is, everything in their lives as children and adolescents was centered on religion and connected to it. Martha, an African-American widow, was one who said, "I was raised in the church." In her case, being raised in the church meant growing up amidst the activities of a large Baptist church in Millerville where her maternal grandparents belonged. She had just returned from a visit to that church the week before our interview. She now lives in Laurelford but had attended a wedding in her childhood church and was clearly delighted to have seen everyone from that religious community. "What a good feeling, it was just like being home again, really, that's what it amounted to." Religion was "very important" and regulated her life during childhood and adolescence. On Saturday the entire family prepared meals for Sunday and completed household chores. Martha spent all day in church on Sundays from Sunday school to formal worship, then had dinner at home (no radio allowed, she told me emphatically), after which people would visit, friends would come in; she could read and talk, then back to the church on Sunday evening. At bare minimum, "Wednesdays too" were spent in religious activities, at least in the evening when there often was a prayer meeting or other events. "Every weekday had a plan, a purpose." Her friends and the friends of her family all were religious people. "When I was coming along, religion was very different." Religious involvement was the entire way of life for the family during the youth of five other older adults. This did not seem to be as much a cohort or gender issue, but seemed to be a function of the overarching and welcome reach of membership in particular congregations. Other elders, two black women, two white women, and one white man, had also grown up in the church. The denominational affiliations were Protestant and mainline in five instances, quasi-mainline for the sixth person.

Others not raised in the church had some powerful experiences during childhood and adolescence—ones that changed their adult lives years later. Gail, 63, recounted that she had a calling to be a minister as early as fourteen. "I knew that's what God had in mind for me. But the churches didn't believe in women ministers at that time. It's not much better now, but it is a little." She couldn't act upon the call as a young woman, but she knew clearly this was something she should do one day. Gail's maternal grandmother had the greatest influence on her beliefs. "She just always believed that no matter what happened, that God was going to be there, and it was going to work out. . . . She was so peaceful. She was always at peace with herself. And I took that to be, because of her belief in God, and He was always going to be there to help her."

Most of the elders were not so immersed in their religions during childhood and throughout young adulthood. They did, however, participate along with their families with mothers leading the way, in the weekly and seasonal observances of their faith. They also were aware of the parallel but "side" activities that were also part of religious involvement—special prayer groups, doing work for the local congregation and occasionally the national organizations, providing room and board for newcomers or visitors—the hands-on, "in-kind" services their families contributed to their religions and to local congregations. This consistent and regular participation is the bedrock of socialization, and even though it was normative or expected of people during the first four decades of the 1900s, the consequence of that participation was that it marked a clear path for faith in adulthood and late life. It's not that the people in the study grew up as saints or that they even think of calling themselves particularly saintly even today, but the precepts, practices, and vocabularies of faith were taught conscientiously by mothers, and it was instilled in them that there were sound ways to be faithful to religious beliefs and good reasons for striving to be so. Though some might later turn to occasional and sporadic worship, or come to substitute ritualistic participation for meaningful involvement, on the whole the group illustrates the maxim that you can only learn what is placed and practiced by you and others around you, and that the most durable practices begin in families or in congregations where families are enfolded.

GENDER AND CHILDHOOD RELIGIOUS SOCIALIZATION

Gender distinctions were most frequently noted by Jewish and Roman Catholic women in the study. The socialization to religion within these orthodox or more conservative forms of faith, as well as the prevailing cultural traditions and definitions of roles and statuses for girls and boys, meant that the formative experiences of men and women had been different. This was not mirrored in the opportunities for secular educational attainment, which was much less linked to gender for the Jews in this sample than was true for their Christian counterparts. In other words, one of the oldest members of the study had earned one of the first baccalaureates in chemistry among Connecticut women. She had, however, missed the opportunity to learn Hebrew and had always participated in an Orthodox shul. Thus, her religious participation was described as meaningful but also as separate from that of men her own age and of men in her own family. Despite the distinctive pathways for boys and girls in terms of religion socialization, for her there had not been a carryover to the expectations and opportunities for her secular education.

Others had experienced gender differences in religious socialization. Lucy terms the Hebrew she was taught as "minimal. . . . He [her father] didn't have much time for me. My sisters got a little bit more of the training, and the focus was more on boys. I went to the Jewish Community—that kind of thing—once a week. Sunday school once a week. I really don't remember a lot of that. It was not enough. So, whatever came to me, came—I don't know—somehow by osmosis or just coincidental or reading a lot—whatever. I learned more as I could by myself." The women spoke in objective ways about this experience and did not appear to be embittered about the gender differentiation that was part of their religious life. She continues, "I think keeping the practice was kind of like automatic. It was never forced. I think what I enjoyed very much is that my house carried the tradition by very open hospitality, and when it came to holidays or when it came to the Sabbath, you never knew who was going to be eating with us. It was a big plus. It was something that I feel, to this day, was always interesting. Because we didn't know who my father was going to bring home from synagogue."

CONSONANCE OF FAMILY AND SOCIAL EXPECTATIONS FOR FOLLOWING A FAITH

No matter what social characteristic one poses as crosscutting (race, gender, social class, place), the feature that was universally acknowledged to be the central reason for the practice of faith in youth and early adulthood was that of parental and community expectations. In particular, the strongest source of influence was attributed to mothers and also to other women (aunts, godmothers, grandmothers) in the family circle who directly introduced matters of faith into the life of the child. This makes eminent sense because in generational terms the people in this study were all born before World War II. Even the youngest people had a minimum of two decades of life where the uncertainties and pace of social change did not find a sturdy place to roost in the larger culture. The oldest members of the study as well as the youngest, the 60-year-olds, grew up in a social structure that still featured religion and religious involvement as normative in a way that is unfathomable for most of us at any age today. This taken for granted feature of religion would change most dramatically for the tail-enders of the baby boom, but even among this Boomer cohort as a whole (1946–1964), the normative structure had not been significantly altered until much later in their life course. Those born before World War II experienced many profound social changes that lagged sufficiently behind and did not significantly alter folkways surrounding religious belief and behavior in the U.S. until many years later, perhaps beginning at the end of the 1950s and culminating at the end of 1960s. This cauldron of social change in the overarching cultural norms and folkways surrounding religion and sacred observance occurred well after people in the study and of their generation of older adults donned adult roles and statuses. Thus, the adult orientation to religion followed on logically and socially without major disjunctures or disruptions in the deeply entrenched faith that had been instilled and reinforced during adulthood.

Maxine was raised in the Dutch Reformed church, "It was absolutely taken for granted. We were born into it." She attended Sunday school and services, participated in choir, "But it was taken for granted. You didn't not go." Though her neighborhood had Catholic and Jewish families and she had close friends from those faiths, she emphasizes that many of her friends were found within this religious community; "we sort of grew up together. We were like a whole pack of brothers and sisters."

Describing what religion meant to him as a younger adult, Phillip shrugged his shoulders slightly and said, "Well, it was just part of the program. I mean, you expected to do it. You expected to have it. And it was partly social but also educational, I always thought. It was a little stimulating educationally, partly history. I mean, that's what appealed to me too."

Early socialization is a cornerstone for commitment in late life. People recalled how religion was fitted into their lives as children in a way that was seamless for most. Religion was one with life—integrated normatively and in such an encompassing way by other social institutions in the community that they came to expect it of themselves just as it was expected of them by others. Religion was not understood as a discretionary choice or one which necessitated great thought as to why and wherefore. Though religions themselves formed a hierarchy reflecting differential evaluations by society and culture, the thought of not learning about or then exercising a religious frame of reference or orientation to life was as unthinkable then as it is today for children to be without the opportunity to learn and exercise the audio and visual links to mass media and computer technology as dominant frames of reference for their own orientation to social life. The frames of reference for social interaction are arguably on qualitatively different substantive levels, for the expectations have shifted away from questions of ultimate concern (religion) to issues of proximate information (media). Thereby hangs a tale about the passing of social worlds defined by generational status and the foreshadowing of "saturated" (Gergen, 1991) or "protean" (Lifton, 1993) new selves that will cast doubt on Wordsworth's heretofore trustworthy insight and claim that the child is father to the man. Put simply, the anchored identities characteristic of the older adults in this study, and the quasi-anchored identities of the Boomer generation, are likely not to be found among today's post-modern children and young adults.

Lest we get too far ahead of ourselves, the repetition and reinforcement of participation in religion throughout childhood is a crucial factor in understanding how older adults described their involvement in late life. Many years ago Robert Coles interviewed elderly respondents in New Mexico. One elder, Mrs. Garcia, talked about the value of habits in old age. "Habits are not crutches; habits are roads we have paved for ourselves. When we are old, and if we have done a good job, the roads last and make the remaining time useful: we get where we want to go, and without the delays we used to have when were young" (Coles, 1975, p. 39). A quarter of a century later, this remains an apt description with respect to religious involvement for a majority of people in this study.

CHAPTER THREE

The Folkways of Prayer in Late Life

"So, like they say, you thank the man for everything He's done for you—giving you sight, giving you your mother and your father, and being around, buying food for you and putting clothes on your back."

The term "folkways," an important concept derived from anthropology and widely used by anthropologists and sociologists, is defined as the customary ways of doing things within a culture and society (Sumner, 1940). There are folkways of dress, food, language, and social interaction, and there are what I call here, folkways of faith, customary ways of "doing" religion, of acting to honor the sacred. William James (1929) was perspicacious in grasping the psychological and experiential range or "varieties of religious experience," but it was the early or classical anthropologists and sociologists writing in the late 1880s into the early 1900s who theorized and demonstrated empirically that cultures and societies formulate norms and transmit customary behaviors pertaining to what is sacred to their members. From Marx's characterization and explicit derogation of religion as "the opium of the people" to Freud's judgment about its illusory and deceptive nature (1964), followed decades later by Ellis's (1985) brief that questions the psychological fitness of those subscribing to religious beliefs, even these severe critiques contain backhanded acknowledgments of the powerful force that religious folkways and norms exert on social structure and individual lives.

Folkways of faith are the usual, or what we may call the taken-for-granted practices, surrounding what is sacred or religious. Folkways of faith are typical, everyday ways of living some part of the many elements of religious belief. Thus, folkways reflect what is typical for a group rather than what is idiosyncratic or unique for a few. Though other social and historical forces influence folkways of faith both in substance and in form, the presence of social institutions of faith, that is, religions, as well as folkways of religious faith are virtually universal across cultures and societies. Indeed, in this chapter, customary ways of doing religion as well as the salience and meaning of religion are identified from the accounts and descriptions of older adults and from the participant observations that were a feature of the long-term care subset of the study as a whole. The most important of these customary ways of doing things relative to a definition of what is sacred, of keeping the faith, include but are not restricted to the following: regular participation in formal worship services; some participation in the array of congregational or collective activities; and, what emerges as most significant, the many private acts of reverence and piety that engage people on a daily or weekly basis far away from the public, formal, and visible participation within a congregation. The primary religious folkway for older adults, the way they keep their respective faiths as part of their lives and identities, is through the activity of praying. Prayer is followed by other ways of keeping faith, such as displaying and using a range of religious symbols and items; participation in formal worship and in devotional groups that are informal as well as formal; engagement with other activities of a congregation or of the faith as a whole; financial support of a congregation or denomination; and for a notable, if small group, encounters or special experiences with nature as well as the mystical experiences described by even fewer people.

PRAYER AS A PRIMARY FOLKWAY OF FAITH AND RELIGION

In this sample as a whole, the folkways surrounding prayer do not vary clearly or strongly according to standard, social scientific categories that generally work effectively to demarcate social differences. Gender, ethnicity, social class, kind of residential setting, health status, living alone or living with someone else, did not, for example, separate those who prayed from those who did not pray. Daily prayer was described and recounted as the most meaningful way of connecting with the divine and the sacred for most people in the study. Recent loss of a loved one, and beliefs about the transcendent dimension of religion, did distinguish to a minor degree the majority of those who prayed from the smaller but discernible group who no longer prayed. However, even among the latter group, death of a loved one and some waning of salience of religious belief most often discriminates with respect to the quality and meaning attached to the prayer experience at the moment. In two cases, where losses were translated into what Thomas (1999), following up on Myerhoff's earlier observations (1980), calls, quarreling with God, the relatively recent death of a loved one was related to dropping prayer entirely from one's folkways of faith.

Religious affiliation slightly influenced prayer in terms of the form of language used to talk with God; that is, among Catholics the standard, formal prayers were more likely to be used than prayers with original phrasing. Overall, the nominal religious preference or denominational label within a religion was not associated with the practice of prayer or the significance individuals attached to praying. The familiar verses of standard prayers were used by most older adults in the study, although saying prayers by using original words was almost equally widespread. Indeed, among those who prayed regularly, 38 people in the study, there were two sharply defined groups: one that was more inclined to the use of standard prayers, and used them; and one that was less inclined to use standard prayers, and made up their own prayers. The smallest group used both standard prayers and their own words. People who used standard prayer were reassured of following faith by using those traditional words daily and in saying them alone or with others in the more occasional setting of both informal and formal devotion or worship. Among Roman Catholics in the study, saying the rosary, an extended form of prayer, was discussed as a much anticipated and important experience that gave them an opportunity to pray and also one that elicited responses to other human beings. For Roman Catholics in long-term care facilities, saying the rosary weekly with others was a very special time during their week as well as a time that evoked fond and positive memories of earlier life and past experiences. Marie, for example, noted that if she missed this group prayer, "It leaves an empty feeling, you know. You watch the five-thirty rosary. There's something else going on. No rosary? Oh, geez. I go in the bedroom and I turn my chair around, and we say it to ourselves. There's something missing [otherwise]." For two other Roman Catholics in long-term care facilities, saying the rosary did not spark particular interest or encourage their attendance and participation.

In Judeo-Christian religious traditions, prayer may occur as part of a public, group activity (the prayer may be coordinated or, as in some traditions, may proceed at a self-defined pace within the group) or prayer may occur as a separate, private, individual interaction. Respondents in the study had much to say about how important praying was to them, although for eight people prayer was not a folkway of faith in their present lives. With respect to prayer, the chief themes that emerged from analysis of interviews were these: prayers are offered at least once daily; prayers are characterized as talking with God, but there is some difference in the kinds of talks that one initiates—that is, prayers vary in terms of specific content; the language of prayer may be uniform or original; and, prayers are implicitly and sometimes explicitly differentiated from prayers said in larger groups, including collective, formal worship services. Each of these points will be discussed with reference to specific examples from the study.

PRAYERS AS TALKS WORTH HAVING EVERY DAY

Prayer is the most frequently mentioned form of religious behavior among older adults in the study. For 38 people, prayer is offered on a daily basis, and is described by them as a multifaceted form of behavior. The meaning of prayer varies among the older adults but it is deemed important and is conscientiously practiced by a majority of those interviewed. Jean's statements that "prayer is important; if prayers are not answered, you go on," and her daily time for prayer, "morning and night," are typical of the group. When she first retired she attended mass daily. Now her private prayer twice a day suffices, along with mass on the Sabbath. Martha, 74, describes herself as "on my knees every day." She recounts time spent previously in a nursing home about a year before our interview when "I stayed in bed, but got on my knees in bed, and prayed every night. I was brought up like that. And you know what bothers me? Even though I brought my children up like that I don't think they take the time to pray."

Margaret, who lives at White Pines, said that she prayed "Every day. Several times a day. Inwardly. That's right. They're in my own words. I have my own little prayers that I say. And I pray for my parents, who are in Heaven, and my relatives—all of them that are in Heaven. And I pray for my family—my husband—and every one that has gone to Heaven." Margaret keeps religious items in her room. "Oh, yes. I have my cross and I have my prayer books. . . . I think most of my prayer books—I love those. I guess most of them were printed before Vatican

II [laughs]." She does not, however, consult these prayer books in order to pray. Many of those who prayed were like Alice, 84, who used "some of the prayers and some my own. I say, 'I'm praying for this one or that one,' grandchildren and everything. And to myself, while I'm falling asleep." Others like Anne, 77, said "You know, I say my prayers and everything, every day in my own way. . . . Well, actually, at least not a whole long length of time every day. Sometimes it's short, maybe 10 or 15 minutes in the morning, 10 or 15 minutes at night. But, I mean, there is a prayer at least once a day. . . . I'm not much on formal prayers. A lot of it is, you know, thoughts and meditation and kind of combining things, or things I may be experiencing in the day I turn into a prayer."

Most people seemed to distinguish immediately and implicitly between praying in a place of collective worship and what they actually meant by praying, which was saying own prayers in private settings outside and separate from places of worship. This is interesting because we generally understand that sacred worship services involve prayers offered by celebrants or clergy, alone or in concert with the congregation as a mainstay of liturgy. However, only a few elders connected weekly service or worship to what they meant by prayer. The institutional, collective, or liturgical prayer of formal services involves praying, but is perceived and defined as a substantively different activity within a markedly different setting. Prayer in the setting of formal services was explicitly referred to by some as "reading from books," or as following along and on cue providing responses to clergy who were conducting the service. Remarks made by James, 74, illustrate the preference for prayers in one's own words as ways to bring others into the communication in a unique and special way. His comments also suggest that the institutional setting is conducive to a different kind of praying. "I'm pretty much in my own words. I used to pray with the, you know, words we were taught. But I think I'm more individual now because I've got so many people to pray for and they got, [chuckles] all my nephews are married, and they've got about five kids apiece, my great-nieces and nephews, you know. And you've got to include them, you've got to. So it takes me a half an hour to pray, for crying out loud. . . . I take them . . . and I pray for each one as an individual. I get closer that way when I pray as an individual. If I say the rosary or something—I mean, I will say the rosary, but to me that was fine when I wasn't here, when I was away from this place, Chelsea Court. But now I feel I'm equipped to pray the way I want to pray. And that's what this has done for me here because it's always available. I mean, you can always go to church [mass is regularly held in the long-term care facility's chapel] and pray. You can always talk to somebody [God] that way."

Patrick, 86, stated that "I pray a lot now that I'm sick, and, oh, I'm not going to live too long. I know that now . . . I use the prayers that were taught to me. If you can't pray, I don't know what you do." I asked if television with its various programs helped. "Oh yeah, that helps," he said, "but you can't watch all day. When I've got the book there [he points to a Bible] and I pray—I've got two other booklets over there," he says that he gains a sense of purpose and some peace. He sometimes uses a rosary for his own prayer, but is more likely to say the rosary weekly as part of a small group. "Some days there's only myself and her [pastoral care team member who visits the nursing home]. And I said to her, 'You shouldn't have to come up here just for one.' She says, 'I'll come up here if there's just one. I love to say the rosary and you say it with me.' Some of the people don't answer the prayers, you know. But I answer them all because my mother, when I was a little bit of a kid, well, my mother. . . . Every single night [she taught him a new prayer] and then we started the rosary and I learned. She taught me the rosary backwards." This last statement was said with good humor as other than the introductory prayers, a rosary is a circle of prayers with a standard variation that makes for a logical forwards and backwards, hence a sequence that is not difficult to master. As one person remarked, rosary beads help with the counting of prayers, not so much with the "thoughts that go into the praying." One important point is laced throughout the interviews as a whole and is reiterated by Patrick: Learning to say prayers is strongly attributed to early socialization and the instruction received from mothers.

THE PURPOSE OF PRAYER: TALKING WITH GOD

Prayer was defined by many as a person's talking with God or connecting with and communicating with a divine force in a private setting. Joan, 89, was straightforward about prayer as a daily commitment. "It keeps me up an hour, maybe, talking to God, [laughs] . . . but I pray to God and say what I have to say." Others like Ruth, 96, a resident of Maple Way, prayed by reading from a book. This kind of private prayer, using books, was the exception not the rule, but it is interesting to note that for Ruth reading from a book may be related to the fact that she does not have a personalized God in mind as the recipient of the prayer. "I pray to a God, but it's hard to believe that there's anyone—that there is a person." Most elders perceived prayer as different ways of talking with God; the variation was in their understanding of God as either personalized and responsive, or a more abstract yet divine force. This dichotomy followed nominally religious lines in that Jews were less likely than their Christian counterparts to invoke the image of a personalized God, but the sample size is too small for this tendency to be more than suggestive of a more substantial difference. The manner in which elders envisioned and imagined the listener to prayers, God, follows along lines that are suggestive of both religious influence and the influence of contemporary cultural typifications in the U.S. that portray the divine or God as an understanding and sympathetic listener. This image of God as filling the role of a listener is prevalent among older adults.

Books, prayer books, core sacred texts, as well as devotionals of all sorts were read by many in the study, generally on specific occasions, but in some instances, devotionals were a daily mainstay. However, there was a distinction drawn between the activity and nature of interaction involved with reading and the activity and interaction involved in praying. As one of the oldest members of the sample said after describing her prayer practice, "I don't know anything special I do. I read my Bible. I used to start, I don't know how many times I've read the Bible through. I've got marks in the Bible every time I read it, so when I know a chapter, I mark it. And then I'll get through and then I'll go back and maybe start with Genesis and read through again. Genesis or Matthew or songs. I don't know. I don't pick out anything special. I just read. And every time I read it, I won't say every time, but many times I read it I think, 'I didn't see that before.'"

Another characteristic shared by the 38 people who prayed was the widespread belief in the value and power of prayer. Val, a resident of Daphne Lane, fully expresses this in her remarks. "I always loved to pray. I believe in prayer." When asked about the most important aspect of prayer, she replies, "I can't answer that; I don't know. I know it gives you a nice feeling. I believe in prayer." She continues by saying that prayers are powerful and helpful, "Oh, it eases the pain and all." She remarks that both physical and emotional pain are eased through prayer. Val adapts her repertoire of standard prayers by using different prayers for different situations. "I always say a little prayer that Irish priests taught me, 'Holy Mary, Mother of God, Remember me and pray for me.' I always say that. And when I can't sleep, I repeat, 'Jesus, Jesus, Jesus,' and I fall asleep." She teaches prayers to others around her, residents and staff alike. "Oh, when the opportunity arises I tell them. In fact, we had a nun here that was a social worker, Sister Agnes. She always used to say, 'Val, do you have a prayer for us?' And she had to have an operation. She had a tumor on her brain. So I told her the prayer, 'Holy Mary, Mother of God, Remember me and pray for me.' She wrote it down. She went to have her operation and it [the tumor] was benign." Val was once an avid reader and misses reading the Bible. "I'm blind in one eye, and being paralyzed, I can't hold a book. I can't turn the pages. But I used to read anything I could get my hands on before . . . everything, anything I could get my hands on. I love to read. I can't do it now. I could read it but I can't handle the book." She also describes religious music which she loves—"it's soothing and it's really a prayer." The prayerful qualities of music were observed as important by some others in the study.

KINDS OF PRAYER, TIMES FOR PRAYER

Prayers of Gratitude and Appreciation

Barbara, 79, offers prayers regularly. As she puts it, "I don't always get what I pray for but I pray for it anyhow. Well, first of all, I want God to know I appreciate all he does for me, because all my family, including my niece and her husband and my sister-in-law, everybody's good to me and maybe I don't deserve it but they are." She prays, "before I go to bed and when I get up in the morning."

There were those who preferred to pray in the morning, those who favored the evening, and some who prayed both morning and evening. There were also a few for whom prayer was like breathing, a continuous, nonvocalized talking; in postmodern imagery, a datastream to the divine. Grace, 61, prays gratefully, though as she understands it, the normative standard about timing of prayer may be different from her practice. "Yes. In the morning. Mostly you're supposed to say your prayers at night: Thank the man upstairs for letting you make it through the day and be able to eat. Hope to see another day. . . . We don't only have one special person to pray for. Pray for everybody."

Beth, 71, says prayers privately every day and also during a portion of formal services. "Oh, I'm just thankful so many times, and I do pray in bed lots of times. . . . I have a whole list of people. We have silent prayer at church regularly. . . . But mostly I wake up in the morning and I'm just grateful for another day [laughs]. I say, 'Thank you, God.' And things are beautiful. I do say 'please' a lot, too, for things to go well. I worry about [a particular family member] that he's doing well." Prayer for her is a substantial feature of faith: "I guess you have faith if you pray to God. You have to have faith. He doesn't always answer prayers. But I think knowing it's there, having faith gets you through all the time."

Maxine, 77, does not offer formal prayers but does offer her own words of gratitude every day. "Oh, I am aware. Rather than formal prayer, I am aware every day, and every day I say, 'Thank you,' if it's not a specific thing. Now I do not request anything because I can remember requesting that I can stick around while my mother was here so I could take care of her. Well, she died in 1984. And then, there was one other thing, the last one was—you know, I wouldn't mind sticking around until the Millennium. But that was a very casual thought." She adds that her informal prayers are "Just thanks, thanks. There's so much to be thankful for. The home. The Lord has taken care of the home, kept it safe during storms when we've had—there are trees all around and He kept us safe. Home is important to me and a lot of members of my family."

Prayers of Petition

Requests for Guidance and Fortitude.   For Rose, 68, prayer is part of seeking guidance. I ask through the translator if Rose prays during the day at all. "She says that you don't need to be in a special place or circumstance or moment to talk to God. That you can be anywhere, at any time, and talk to God. She says that she doesn't do it all day, all the time. Sometimes when she feels bad, she needs help because she has a problem, or somebody has a problem. She will ask Him for His guidance and for His help, and she also prays to Him." Mostly Rose prays using her own words, not the standard versions of prayer. There were a few others who spoke of "bringing things to prayer," "praying over" an issue, or of "carrying it to God through prayer." Seeking the benefit of counsel through prayer was an important theme for some older adults and part of the purpose and content of prayer.

Wanda, 83, prays regularly. "Well, I know I have to keep going and when I say my prayers I pray just for strength [chuckles]. Just to get through it [life every day]—just for strength." Others agreed that praying was a source of strength; they received an intangible but real sense of fortitude that helped them to work through tough situations and to find the physical energy and psychological balance to keep doing what needed to be done in their lives. From this perspective, praying may be viewed as a conversation that permits active coping. It is an interaction that permits recognition of difficult issues posed in late life and it is a long-familiar activity that simultaneously acknowledges the challenges confronted and the reason for the person to keep moving through the day. Here prayer is a trunk line for communication with the divine. The messages are modified by specific situations and circumstances and the line is always open.

Requests for Specific Help or Intervention. One person described prayer as giving her a sense of satisfaction and of autonomy, although it did not seem to be changing a serious health problem. "And that [praying] makes me feel good. I feel that I did something. I know it's such a good feeling. . . . I pray for my children. I mean, there's no use, I used to pray that this would get better [an immobilized arm, the result of a stroke]. If I could use my finger, I could use a walker or something. But I'm giving up hope [that prayer will alter this]." This person was one of less than a handful of people whose prayers were requests for specific help. It is also a rare instance of someone who used prayer to request a concrete change in health. Some people in the study petitioned for favorable outcomes in the lives of others, particularly family members and loved ones, but even those requests were usually phrased in general terms. The pattern of shying away from use of prayer to petition for definite outcomes in health was interesting. Prayer seems to be understood widely as the kind of conversation that is not the place to ask for specific assistance with health. Though guidance in the search for strength and fortitude make up a good part of the daily conversation talking with God, God, the ultimate listener, is not typically understood or characterized as a super-sized ombudsman or a supreme problem-solver. Prayer may render valuable assistance to individuals in coping with particular problems, but the power of prayer seems to reside in the act of formulating the words cogently and with sincerity by the individual, much more than in any actual, literal expectation a person might have about receiving an answer or a solution.

Douglas, 73, noted that prayer in general was all about asking for needs to be met. "I pray in the morning, very seldom at night. But in the morning because I generally wake up, it's quiet, I will pray . . . they're just standard, traditional, Our Father, the Hail Mary. I might throw in a few quickies on the side. But like people say, you're always asking for something. You're always—you know, you're asking God for something all the time. . . . You're petitioning him for—he's not to blame. So you're actually asking him for something that he's not, you know, he doesn't make you sick. He's not the one that wants you to be sick; he's not the one that wants you to be hurt, which you're always asking him for something. You should be able to thank him." Douglas also follows a daily devotional which contains short prayers. "There's batches every day . . . it's two minutes." He reads them conscientiously.

Marie, 90, prays in "my own [words] except, if something comes up and my children have to go under for a test or something, I would pray for them, things like that [chuckles]. And I'll say, 'Dear God, forgive me, but I'm begging again.' " She recalls a time in her life when many people said prayers over her as she moved in and out of consciousness with extensive and critical injuries from a fire. "And they would say prayers over me [in the hospital] when I wasn't able to come out of [unconsciousness]." She sees and credits medicine as having worked hard to restore her to health, but the indelible scarring that remains from the trauma and the vivid memories that the scars evoke even years later are tangible reminders for her of all the prayers that others once said for her.

Donna, 62, prays daily, though these days she's not very conscientious about attending weekly services. "Oh, a lot. Yeah, that I do [laughs]. That I do. I have to say my prayers, and most of the time it's about me and my family—to take care of them and stuff, which He does pretty well." She prays, "In my own words, very silently, at night, usually just before I go to sleep."

Julia, 75, has a wider perspective on prayer, though like others she has used prayers of petition. "Well, I never asked for anything, I only ask for big things, like peace within my family. My granddaughter asked me last year, 'What do you pray for?' I said, 'I always pray for the same thing.' She said, 'What?' I said, 'Peace.' She said, 'You pray for peace!' [laughs] You know, she'd pray for a new bicycle or something. But, you see, she's too young to understand. So, I guess the main thing is when different people are sick, and a death in the family, or something like that. But I don't pray for little things. . . . I use my own words, usually. Or I'll say the Lord's Prayer or something like that. But usually, I use my own words. I talk, you know, I talk to God. That's about it, I think."

Prayers Foregone

Amidst this largely prayerful group were eight people who did not pray daily or regularly. Max, 74, says, "I used to pray, but since my wife passed away, I don't." He emphasizes that this is not a rejection of his religion, but he does not wish to have these talks and no longer prays. Others like Edward, 60, a widower, have changed their practice of prayer, "I pray now and then. I don't pray as much as I used to." Indeed, he had dropped off considerably from what he described as his earlier practice of daily prayer. "I think the religion helped me get through a lot of things when [his wife] was sick. Before she was sick I never really thought about it but it seemed like with the religion we came closer. Church, praying, we used to pray together [at home] ask for help and intercession. If there was no religion, it would have been just blah. It was something that we shared."

Alex, 76, doesn't pray much at all but does read sacred and religious books and other materials. "No, I wouldn't say I pray. But I read the books. Every word has a meaning to me. It isn't that I read and it doesn't have any sense to me. When we were young and when you learn to read the prayers, one word is the same as the other one, and that's about it. But to me, you know, I read and I say, 'What am I saying? To whom am I praying? What am I praying to?' " The critical aspects of thinking and reading are valued more highly by him than the dialogical aspects of praying. Others, like Phillip, 93, were succinct. He describes his praying as "not that much."

This group of eight also includes four people who said that they did not pray independently either formally or informally outside the institutional or formal setting of worship. For example, Libby, 74, only prays as part of larger formal worship, "Well, if I'm in the synagogue, I read the prayer book." The three other women who do not pray are a bit more ambiguous about prayer. Lucy, 76, does not pray though in all other respects she keeps her faith. "No, I can't say I do. I think of God and so forth, but I don't set aside any time to pray. No . . . I don't set the time for that." Later when we talk about religious items in her home I notice Sabbath candles, and she confirms again that "for myself" there is no prayer, but she does do "Mostly the blessings on the candles. That's what I continue to do, will never stop, I hope. That's it. I mean, I don't open a book and start to read prayers, no." Thus with respect to what Myerhoff (1980) has called the "domestic" elements of religion that Judaism embraces, particularly with respect to the Sabbath blessing which is a weekly observance held at home and shaped by short standard prayers, it is clear that Lucy says these prayers and sees them as integral to the larger milieu of Judaism. The Sabbath prayers are domestic, but they are also important as cultural as well as religious links to a faith.

Continuous Prayers

There is a complexity to prayer that is often neglected when prayer is treated, as it is often characterized, as a unitary event or a single act. The extended example that follows comes from Gail, 63. She is a minister and unsurprisingly she prays. However, as she describes how she prays, the continuous and significant part it has in her life as a person, not only as a minister, becomes evident. Like other people in the study, she emphasizes the dialogical or relational component with God as central to prayer. Yet for her and for a few others prayer is much more than a daily check-in with the divine. "Even as I speak, I'm praying for the right thing. Constantly. I don't think it's—I think prayer is almost with me a never-ending kind of thing. And I pray for thanksgiving. I pray for things that I need. I pray for other people. It's kind of like any time I think about anything, I can say a prayer. 'Well, thank you, Lord, for that.' You know, 'Lord, please help.' If I go in a store and I see somebody who is not necessarily handicapped [physically] . . . someone who appears to be out-of-state with God. You know, swearing or cursing—just profane—a number of profanities [are] coming out of them . . . I pray for that person more than I would for somebody who was on crutches, because that person on the crutches might have more understanding than the person who [profanes]. I pray for everything. I pray for my car [laughs]. I pray for everything. And it works, you know." After describing some instances of prayer she adds, "Prayer is—sometimes, you know, I think that people think you have to—well, for me—I don't always get in the prayer position, like you see with the praying hands and you've got to be on your knees and you need to be in church. To me, prayer is communication with God, and I need to be with him all the time. Like in meetings. Wherever I'm sitting, and I'm not talking I'm generally, I'm praying."

Pauline, 87, prays daily in her own words and observes that "It seems as though God gives us words to say. They just come to me. I don't have no certain time to pray. I pray when I get up in the morning, when I go to bed at night. No special time. And I think about—like, during the day, to myself, God is good. And I use the word 'blessed.' Not 'lucky.' I'm not lucky. I'm fortunate. I'm blessed to be as well as I am." She also "prays over" other matters. "And I love people, you know. At least six persons have died since I've been here [her apartment]— good friends of mine—and it just did something to me. My heart goes out, I'm not only interested in my own folks. If I know of a person, just like the different accidents, it affects me to the extent that I have to pray over the matter. . . . Well, that's what makes me what I am—my faith. Okay, I'm a strong believer. My minister says, 'When you pray, if you don't believe in prayer, it don't do you any good.' That's what he says. So, I agree. You pray. You ask God for different things. If you don't believe that He will do it [answer], it don't benefit you." Later she reiterates this perspective. "I believe that if you pray to God for certain things, and you mean it from your heart, He will answer. But as I was saying before, if you don't believe in it, you're just wasting your time if you don't believe in it. You're just trying to test God with something, but God don't fail. And if you believe that He don't fail, it does you good." In the high-rise apartment building where she makes her home, there is a distinctive place-marker on her door. A neighbor and friend made and painted a wooden angel with accompanying words, "Shh. . . . Talking with God," to grace Pauline's doorway.

Another person whose prayers were an almost continuous thread of daily life was Clara, 90. "I pray all the time. I don't have a set prayer hour, some people have. They read the Bible and then they have to have a prayer time. I don't do that. I pray the whole day. And I believe that God will keep bringing things to you, to pray. And many times, I'll be just working around those a little bit, and all of a sudden, somebody will come to me or something will come to me and I'll say, 'Pray for them. Pray for that.' But to sit down, for me to, I used to do that. But for me now [a formal period set aside for prayer would be] just a ritual. . . . I can't stay into a ritual prayer session." Clara also has a prayer list: "I have a prayer list I keep in my Bible. I've got all different names. I've got a list of names. If somebody wants me to pray for them, I'll write their name on that prayer list. Now, I don't go down over that prayer list every day and pray for this one and this one. I just [say] 'I don't know what their need is, I don't know what they should have, but you do. And today, meet their need.' "

Even when people admitted that their own formal religious affiliation and participation had not been continuous throughout life, they often said, like Walter, 70, that prayer had always been part of their daily behavior. "I went through a period where I didn't go to church on Sundays because when you work in a [a particular business], you work until twelve or one o'clock in the morning, and it was very difficult for me to get up on Sunday mornings and go. But I've never—I still pray. And I have a Bible by my bed. It does open, you know." He usually starts praying with a Hail Mary, though he is Episcopalian, and proceeds to add his own prayers, in his own words. He also petitions with prayer. After two serious operations, "I pray for better health. I don't want to be sick. I have a very deep feeling that I don't think that my health condition as it is today is going to take me. I still think I have a few good years left. I have a special prayer. I say 'Oh, dear God, let me live to be seventy-five.' " Indeed, Walter's view is that public prayer and formal observance may not save hypocrites, "You can go into a closet and pray to God and be with God. But I see people that—they consider themselves very religious because they go to church every Sunday, and they put the largest amount of money in the basket, and that sort of thing. But God takes care of the poor people. And I know people that, they're hypocrites. But that doesn't make any difference, because God loves everybody. God gets a kick out of the hypocrites."

Married Couples and Prayer

The experiences described by married couples in their separate interviews do not suggest that their practice of prayer is significantly different from that of older adults who are married (but whose spouses were not part of the study) or from that of those who live alone (single, divorced, or widowed) in terms of the role prayer plays as a folkway of faith. With respect to the five married couples interviewed in the study, in three couples there was a mutually shared engagement with prayer as well as a similar depth of concern and level of involvement with institutional or formal participation in religion. For one of the two remaining couples there was a fundamental agreement about the value of faith and of religious beliefs as important for establishing a "way of life," but the individuals in the marriage had differing perspectives and patterns of involvement with prayer. For another couple, there was minimal engagement both with folkways of faith and in formal participation with religion. In other words, there was a high degree of overlap or agreement on folkways and institutional participation for four married couples, and for one couple a discernible distance had emerged because one person had considerably altered the orientation to religion. In this last couple, one person had not so much become an apostate or dropped previous patterns of interaction; instead there had been a sea change in terms of belief about the divine and about the meaning of the Bible and of the liturgy. This pattern is important although it did not typify the pattern among married couples or among older adults in the study. Another way to put this is that for four of the five married couples, the connection and interaction with religious domains was still jointly framed and each partner, in terms of both their individual identities as well as an identity as part of a married couple, anticipated that this mutually sustained level of engagement would continue in their lives.

Among some of the married elders (whose spouses were not part of the study) there was some discussion about how spouses diverged from beliefs and behaviors that had once been jointly defined and shared, or about longstanding differences that had existed across life with respect to religious values and folkways of faith. One person, whose professional role was that of a minister, noted that the spouse's orientation and behavior differed considerably from the minister's. This example is illustrative of the elasticity within a relationship between two people who have been long-married. A major point here is that even among those presently or formerly married, sharing or being very close to sharing similar religious backgrounds (as in the case of the minister) was a likely source of encouragement for "keeping the faith" as one aged and moved through all of the events of life, but it did not prevent individuals from formulating or practicing their own version of what was needed to keep that faith.

Married couples interviewed in the study, as well as widows and widowers, frequently reported that they prayed together or had prayed together, sometimes regularly as a well-established folkway and sometimes situationally in response to or in recognition of particular circumstances or events that called for thankfulness or petition. For example, Eugene, 82, prays twice a day: "I pray before I go to bed and when I get up in the morning." His practice is often shared by Nora, his wife, at certain times of the day. "Yes," says Nora, "we pray every morning. I pray every morning. Every morning. Sometimes during the day, there are books that I have in the living room, and there are magazines back there, and I pick them up and say a couple prayers. And it's great satisfaction. And if there's something on my mind, to bother me, I say a prayer." Nora also provides some direct evidence of how powerful prayer can be in efforts to change other aspects of behavior. Speaking about her success in giving up cigarette smoking, she says that during that time of life, "I never prayed so much in my life. And I was working at the time. I was working [at a large corporation] and there were several people around in different departments that smoked. They would light up, and I would see them—right in front of me. [Laughs] And I would see them and I would gaze at it for a few minutes, and then I would say my prayer, and that kept me going. So, I can tell you now that if it weren't for the prayer and the faith of the good Lord, I would never have gotten through it. It took me a whole year-and-a-half to do it."

Andrew, 92, says this about prayer: "I have felt that prayer was really beneficial. You learn that there are others besides you who need the help of prayer, and a great many times the prayers are answered without hesitation. It's been a source of not only inspiration, but a real benefit in what prayer has given to me." His wife, Lydia, 89, says, "I've found that happening when I've had—I've said a prayer for something that was worrying me, and I find as time goes on, that these things turn out the way I wanted them to. I have faith that those prayers that I have said have helped to bring it about. So, there are several occasions when things that worried me so, and I didn't know what to do about it—by having that prayer as a basis for some consolation, maybe we can call it that—it turned out that things did change the way I wanted them to, and I really had faith that the prayer really had something to do with it."

Sally, 79, and her husband, Hank, 80, say the rosary together and also as Sally states, "I say all my prayers in the morning and at night. . . . My [prayer] books are falling apart." She takes one off a nearby bookshelf to show me and describes a visit she made to a local religious retailer to see if this particular prayer book could be reordered. "When I went to that religious store," she was told that the prayer book could not be replaced. "The only thing they told me to use is Scotch tape. It's such a beautiful prayer book. The lady looked at it and she smiled. She said, 'Why don't you use it sometime?' "

Wanda, who is married, but whose spouse was not part of the study, tells much about the ways in which prayer is not only a feature of religious behavior but an important facet of daily life. This is part of the story that Wanda tells. Wanda did not marry until she was "late in life," age 67 in 1984. The couple had a small evening wedding and the bride wore pink. "I never was married before, and the man I married, his wife died, and it was good because it was for companionship and a little security. But now he's got dementia . . . I'm going to keep him home as long as I can, but eventually I'll have to put him in a nursing home." Her husband received the diagnosis about two years prior to the interview. Until two years ago, her husband had been very active (walking, swimming). Though they had lived one street over for most of their adult lives, and in terms of propinquity had been neighbors, they had only met through dog walking. "His wife had died and he had a dog and I bought a dog for myself. After I retired I bought a dog and met him through the dogs." They enjoyed many "good years" of married life until the diagnosis of dementia.

Today her direct participation in formal religious activity has diminished. "Well, I just went to mass and I'd go every week but I'd say for the last three years I go very seldom, you know. And now, I can't go. Can't go at all, you know. It's too hard because I have women coming here at night and taking over for me, so I can get a night's sleep. . . . I got them [through] an agency and they come in at eight o'clock and then they stay with him 'til seven in the morning. And that gives me a chance to get some rest because I couldn't take care of this man 24 hours a day; I couldn't do it. And his mind is going more now; he's more confused. And it's going to get worse as time goes. I don't know what's going to go first, the legs or the mind. But one or the other's going to go. And that's when he'll have to go in the nursing home."

She also says something interesting about care—"It's harder taking care of a man." I point out that she cared for her mother for years, and she notes that her mother didn't have dementia, "when the mind goes, that's awful. And he says last night, 'Well, when are we going home?' He says, 'When are we going home?' I says, 'You are home.' 'Well, when are we going home?' You see, this is what's going now, all of this stuff, you know." She describes her marriage and life as "we had thirteen good years—very good. But right now it is very tough, and prayer helps a bit" but she's in such a juggernaut that other involvement with religion is out of the question. Interestingly enough, the religious community has not been forthcoming with much help for her or her husband. She is making a valiant effort, but also knows clearly that she is alone in this or on her own in coming to terms with the many issues that arise daily.

Parts of Wanda's situation are reflected in the lives of other married people in the study. Eighty-nine-year-old Joan talks about her present husband's continued decline in health. He once had a beautiful singing voice, "On Jewish holidays, he would sing in the synagogue—the prayers," but now it is painful to her to know that he cannot remember any of the words and can no longer sing with the ability he once had. Together they have shared a room in a long-term care facility for four years and she tells me that "He's very, very forgetful. He's got these drawers of socks and underwear and pajamas. He doesn't even know where anything is. He looks for his shoes in the drawer. Terrible, terrible thing. It's a terrible thing to see somebody else being like that, too. It's terrible for me, too. I shouldn't look at him. It's very tough."

Given the depressing situation, one might think that religious participation might help her. But she does not attend formal services even though there is a synagogue on site. "I was President of the Hadassah one time. And we joined Hadassah, and we belonged to the B'nai B'rith, and we belonged to all of the societies—Sisterhoods. I was involved in everything. In the synagogue, I was very much involved in [all the activities] at the time. They had parties and things, you know. [They said] 'Joan's going to put it together. Joan's going to do this. Joan's going to do it.' And I did it. And I enjoyed it. If I didn't enjoy it, I wouldn't do it, you know? I was very much involved in the synagogue. He was, and I was, too. Now, I don't go to synagogue. We have a synagogue here," but she had an unsatisfactory set of initial experiences associated with the synagogue and no longer attends. She participates, however, in many of the secular activities within the facility and most particularly enjoys the volunteers who come in to play bridge twice a week. This challenging card game gives her the chance to schmooze and compete at the same time. Both activities are ones that delight her and make life worth living. Her appraisal of her life today is realistic: "I don't have no other choice, you know. My son wanted me to go to Florida, 'There's a beautiful place there, and it's always warm there,' he said. I said, 'I have all my friends here. They come in from Millerville, you know, and they take me out to lunch and we go here, we go there. There's so many things that we could do here that we couldn't do in Florida. Who am I going to meet in Florida?' In a home, you can't meet people—too many. You have to have somebody around. So, I said, 'No. Please, let me stay. Let me go to Samuelson.' And he came up here and he saw it was so nice and clean," that he accepted the choice.

RESIDENTIAL SETTING AND PRAYER

Type of residential setting did not influence the value and salience of praying, nor did it affect the range of prayers offered by older adults.

However, in two interviews, there was a hint of difference resulting from the physical surroundings of long-term care. The physical structure and quasi-public layout of long-term care facilities does not prevent silent, individual prayer. Nor does the presence or absence of dedicated space for formal worship impede private individual prayer. But two people emphasized that they liked to pray "in the quiet" of the building and for them prayers were offered in the hour before dawn or before darkness, hours of quiet in the noisy life of human activity and of the building. The fact that these two people were residents in facilities that had dedicated space for formal religious observance should not be overlooked. Dedicated religious space, valuable in and of itself to the long-term care residents I interviewed, may not be the most suitable or the preferred setting for the private prayer that most people offer daily.

In the long-term care subset, only one person never prayed; two others rejected the word, prayer. Thinking or reflection were the terms they preferred for their daily conversations with the divine. In all respects, elders in long-term care settings were as prayerful a group as those who lived in the community. Even in the confined settings of long-term care, prayer remains one way to continue to speak with your own voice to another, in this case, God, about needs and hopes. After all, the kind of talk one has with God daily is colloquial, and is unimpeded for the most part by the lack of mobility and autonomy that permeates institutional settings. Thus, prayers were said every day at least once a day by all but one long-term care resident.

WAYS OF PRAYING: SUMMARY

The communal celebration which includes formal prayer on the Christian or Jewish Sabbath is described as a qualitatively different experience that is distinct from prayers that are offered every day. In fact, the language used to describe what people take away from attendance is focused on a very different role for the collective experience of religion. Many people reiterated that attending formal worship was something that was "expected," that was a routine, or that was "just natural," a logical extension of earlier socialization. The reason for regular attendance was attached to a different dimension of the religious role, one in which people as members and congregants were primarily passive listeners, and for some limited moments in the service, participants. When older people described their weekly religious participation it was in terms of taking a message away from a cleric's formal remarks, of doing what was expected and deriving some sense that this was better than skipping, and of sharing with others by being present for them as a member of the group. The word prayer was not often used to describe communal worship, and only rarely did people mention that there were portions of formal worship set aside for prayer. Prayer and attendance or participation are perceived as separate facets of religiosity or separate folkways of faith. Yet prayer itself stands out as the most important folkway of faith though virtually all of what is meant by prayer and defined as salient is what we call individual or private prayer. And even here there is a curious twist in that among a very well-socialized group, the form of prayers was just as often expressed in original phrasing as it was dependent on standard phrasing from specific religious traditions. Among those who used standard prayers at least occasionally in daily prayer and for those who said they did not pray except during formal worship, it seemed that the perception or image of God was to a greater degree more abstract and impersonal than it was for those who prayed using their own words.

As noted in the previous chapter, prayers were taught in childhood and youth, initially almost exclusively by mothers at home, followed by formal religious education and greater exposure to a variety of standard, official prayers. Though many if not most elders in the study had their faith's respective prayer books handy or easily accessible in their rooms—often the sacred texts were clearly visible on a shelf in the room where the interviews were completed—most older adults did not make use of such books in daily prayers. Except among a handful, the sacred books were treated as reference tomes to be consulted infrequently.

Another interesting aspect of prayer as a folkway of faith is that only two or three people were aware of the experience that others had prayed or continued to pray for them. The two people who commented directly about knowing that others had prayed for them, linked that awareness to serious health crises they had each faced. Marie and James described themselves as having been aware of people praying for them as they faced long recuperations from difficult and risk-laden procedures. What's interesting is the nearly universal lack of awareness among elders in the study, that they might have been recipients of prayers from others. Despite the fact that nearly everyone in the study was praying daily for many other people, only two were cognizant of having received the prayers of others.

By and large people prayed frequently, and generally these prayers were of gratitude, praise, or petition. Counsel was also sought by a few.

Prayers of petition were generally acknowledged to be primarily for others and infrequently for themselves. Prayers were also understood to be requests that might go "unanswered," or that might be met in ways that were not expected. On the whole, people were not looking for tangible outcomes or literal results. People who mentioned looking for particular, concrete results also noted that they had largely abandoned that tack with respect to praying. To reiterate a major point noted earlier, God was most often understood figuratively and symbolically as a divine listener and less often as a nonpersonified, abstract force. There was also little evidence in this study that older people prayed with some larger, theological perspective in mind.

In *Old Age*, the Jungian analyst Helen Luke (1987, p. 77) discusses prayer as taking the shape of either "necessity" or "beseeching." She draws upon lines from Prospero's epilogue (four of the lines are highlighted below) in *The Tempest* to illustrate the meaning of "necessity."

" 'And my ending is despair,
Unless I am relieved by prayer,
Which pierces so, that it assaults
Mercy itself, and frees all faults.' "

Necessity, as a dimension of prayer, says Luke, is not " . . . begging for a desired result—even when we sincerely add the easily spoken words 'if it be thy will.' The necessity . . . is the kind of prayer that pierces through to the Mercy, where the opposites unite in pardon . . . it reaches beyond every demand for results." Only a few, if any, older adults in the study could be said to offer prayers that reach this level of "necessity" or insight that Luke identifies and connects with prayer. Moreover, if the standard is relaxed a bit to permit inclusion of the Serenity Prayer as it is commonly known (the prayer's authorship is generally attributed to Saint Francis of Assisi), older adults in the study still cannot be said to use this kind of prayer or this level of prayer. The general form and content of prayers is what Douglas, a member of the sample, calls petition and what Luke calls "beseeching." Prayers of beseeching have " . . . many levels . . . and it is very difficult to know ourselves well enough so that we reach beyond all our various longings for ourselves or for others, beyond even the agonized and right human desire to save others from their suffering, or to be released from our own. Even Christ prayed to be spared, but it was not his fundamental desire. That was unshakably to accept the necessity of his unique destiny."

Prayers of petition and beseeching have many levels, and though people acknowledged that they attempted to moderate their expectations about obtaining results, most prayers did not move beyond asking for results. For example, Val, who found prayer meaningful and salient, spoke of once offering a prayer to get results. "I always said, 'I don't know what I would do if my mother died.' The time came where I prayed for her to die because she suffered. She was a good mother." The beseeching prayer, even one for compassion and relief of suffering, is not a prayer "beyond results." Many of the fervent prayers offered by older adults were ones of petition. A few older adults recognized this as a limitation in their own practice of prayer, but many more were simply unaware of other levels of prayer.

In general, the proffered prayers from members of the study were not reflective or what others might term, meditative (LeClercq, 1982; Marinier, 1954). Instead, the prayers were reflexive and were wrapped within familiar forms that had endured from childhood across decades of lives, or in original words that were found to be meaningful. This is, in its own way, a testament to effective socialization and since the practice of praying had not been abandoned or changed, the process of praying remained active and meaningful to individuals. The vocabulary of prayer and therefore the level of prayer as a communication with the divine were robust, but the vocabularies of prayer were limited. Ironically it is this strong tie to earlier socialization that precludes learning other vocabularies of prayer and of imagining different dialogues with the divine even in the face of despair recognized dramatically by Shakespeare and much later alluded to by Luke. Sociologically it is unlikely that functional vocabularies and styles of prayer, prayers carried through a lifetime, modified slightly by Vatican II or the impulse toward inclusiveness, or even of the more direct participation in worship, could be expected to be substantively different in late life than from earlier stages of life. The alternative, reflective prayer, using words to tap into experiences and relate to God on a new level, or as one person phrased it, "finding new ways to put an awareness of God into words," was found and practiced by only a few people. Successful and continuous socialization across life shaped the content and level of prayer among most older adults toward the familiar and the tried and true. That socialization which is directed to keeping the folkways of faith, assures older adults of a stable vocabulary for praying and a largely unvarying but satisfying style of prayer. In this sense, folkways of faith are cornerstones of social identity in late life. However, this successful religious socialization makes limited use of introspection, reflection, and meditation. Thus prayer itself is an important but not fully explored form of interaction with self or other, in this case, God. As Grace put it, "talking with the man upstairs" works for most people in the study, yet as Luke suggests, the potential quality of prayer of connecting people with the transcendent has not yet been reached. This is not a criticism of how people pray; these prayers of beseeching and gratitude are meaningful and are used by most. However, in terms of opening up avenues for adaptation and change in late life, there is ample room for lessons in the language of prayer and for the kind of exploration into the vocabularies of prayer that may lead to reflective as well as reflexive prayer in late life.

The reservoir of meaning that moves people to say prayers daily and to identify it as one of the most significant features of religion in late life may have important ramifications for religious institutions and for social programs. When I consider how many people pray and do so once or twice a day, even in this somewhat special sample, I am reminded of a statement made many years ago by the sociologist Andrew Greeley. During a television panel discussion on problems faced by mainline denominations, Greeley once said that a deficiency among many mainstream religions in the United States, including Catholicism, was that increases in the overall level of education among adherents were not being considered or addressed by religious institutions or clerical leaders. In a similar vein, I suggest that older adults may suffer as a group from being perceived and perhaps stereotyped by religious institutions and clerical leaders as being "nearer to God" than others, and that this attitude is conducive to a benign neglect with respect to educating the old more carefully and consistently into the more reflective aspects of faith. In the realm of prayer, a very significant folkway of faith for pre–World War II–age cohorts, there are well-established practices that can benefit from greater attention by religions and local congregations. Older people in this study are keeping the faith they have practiced, yet religions themselves have not taken their congregants much beyond the level of prayer that is beseeching. And this is precisely the kind of group, regular attendees, consistent financial supporters and members, where new and intellectually challenging aspects of folkways of faith could be introduced. Inasmuch as daily prayer is a positive sign of stability across major changes that individuals confront in aging, it is also a sign that the practices of childhood are deemed sufficient for late life. But what is sufficient is not all that is necessary for growth, particularly for those, including elders themselves, who are concerned with the quality of late life and the potential for learning new ways of moving through that life.

One of the things I found little evidence for, was the use of self-interested prayer, or what some might term the magical use of prayer. To the extent that there were traces that prayer was understood by a few adults, at least in part, as a kind of magical or superstitious activity, it was found in statements offered about the power that words alone might have to resolve, or literally create solutions for real problems. In a social scientific sense, magical use occurs when standard or original prayers are ascribed a power and reality that is less directed toward the transcendent and more toward a wish for a specific outcome or solution. There was little indication that people in the study used or were prepared to take up magical thinking as a substitute for prayer. However, in a few instances a desired outcome was a primary reason for prayer and the divine was called upon or summoned as an instrument to accomplish this end. That does border on magical thinking, yet again, there are only hints of this in a few responses.

Prayer is a powerful way to create meaning and to provide purpose and activity in life. It is a way of keeping the faith with others and in oneself. It is a folkway that has been activated throughout earlier ages and stages of an older adult's life. Perhaps this begins to explain why it is a meaningful, and among this generation of elders in this residentially stable sample, a sustained folkway. Having a voice and using it is an extremely important aspect of self and identity in late life. Prayer is the exercise of one part of that voice and identity. And though it is unusual to see this association, there was at least one 90-year-old who found that the most effective place to pray was on wheels: "Where do I communicate with God better than any place? When I'm out riding in my car, all by myself. I can communicate with God and worship Him better than any place that I know of. I talk to God more when I'm in my car out driving." This sense of privacy as a condition for prayer (Luke, 1995, p. 27) is a predominant theme in the interviews. The portable privacy of automobiles may even be a very good place for prayer.

CHAPTER FOUR

Other Folkways of Faith in Late Life

"Religion is something you carry with you."

OTHER FOLKWAYS OF FAITH: FORMAL PARTICIPATION IN RELIGION

Among the study elders, both the 36 community-dwelling adults and the 15 people residing in long-term care settings, religious participation in worship or in related activities like congregational committee work, service to the faith, and service to the larger civil and secular community were frequently mentioned as important aspects of how tenets of faith were practiced or followed. Many in the sample were active on congregational and denominational committees, and mentioned this in responding to questions about what faith meant in their lives. Robert, 85, opened his remarks this way. "Well, the participating or some of the things I do in church are I'm on the committees, nothing but formal committees. Always secretarial or the treasury, chairman of the committee, and so on. Then, when it comes to the actual, what does the faith do for me, it's this. With Mother, she always taught me gratitude. Every day is a gift. And promise yourself that you'll give thanks to the Lord for the new day, and you'll rejoice in that. And my prayers every day are thankful." This admixture of the instrumental and social dimensions of faith on the one hand, and the expressive and personal dimensions on the other hand, was found in many comments. Beth wryly observed, "Just sacrifice of time. I taught Sunday school and you give a lot of time preparing lessons and things. Time. Boy, do I give time. Midnight oil,

I burn. But no great sacrifice. I think the benefits far outweigh any real sacrifice. Fellowship. The church is giving a lot to us."

Nora, 77, said, "I take away a lot of comfort and—not satisfaction as much as comfort and peace of mind, maybe. Thank God for what we have—oh, yes. That's what I come away with. Yes. Peace of mind. In fact, God knows us as we are. Not ask too much, but be grateful for what we have. And then, support our parish, too, which is very important. Because those priests work very hard to keep our [parish going]. . . . Definitely. If it weren't for that, if I didn't have faith in the good Lord, I wouldn't be anywhere. I mean, I wouldn't be where I am. I have great faith. It keeps me going." This was echoed in Lucy's remarks. "I'm a believer. That's it. To a good degree that sometimes the more questions you have, then maybe the more you get unstable, you're not as firm in beliefs, that never happened to me. I just feel better when I'm sitting in the synagogue, even if I'm not concentrating fully on everything. I just feel better. When I go, I like to be there, I get something out of it." If she were to miss services, she says she would miss "being there." "You know that we read periodically throughout the year, one chapter after another. And it's the sequential kind of thing, and I feel I'm missing something that week. I just enjoy being there. It's not forced at all. I think the sense of identity is most important to understand, and why am I here? And by the grace of God, why am I here? And how can I be a good person? And I think this teaches us that if you study it, you can find out how we can better ourselves and do better to others in the world. That's the way I look at it."

Others concur and note the unique features of collective worship that make it more memorable than all of their daily prayers. Maxine, for example, mentioned the power of music: "Sometimes it can be some special music that is performed. We have an excellent, excellent pianist, organist, choir director. And, this is a singing congregation. And sometimes there is something very special that really shines after the hour or so. [The minister] gives us such wonderful messages. He really allows himself to be spoken through. And because he does that, we are able to be fed. So, we never go away without something. If we keep our hearts open to it. If you're going to go in there with an attitude, maybe you're not going to get anything. But if you're open, you'll get something." If Maxine did not attend, she would miss "Everything. The people. The people. Aside from the spoken word and the music, it would be the people. Because they are my delight. They are my family. Besides my blood family, which is all over the world. But this is my extended family. I would miss them." Clara's perceptions are similar. "Oh, I don't know. I just like the spirit that's in the meetings. That's what I like. There's a free spirit there. Not so much today as they used to be, but there is—there's something about it. I don't know. I believe they live what they teach most of us. Of course, there's always something that I don't agree with." The theme of belonging and finding in regular attendance and participation the indescribable but palpable something special was key. As Anne says, "I go to service, actually, just to kind of, just to kind of feel that love that I think is so important. I don't always go to seek some big major thing or whatever. I just go for comfort and love."

Another way to think about reasons for participating in the religious community and not merely the prescribed formal worship, is related to the survival of that particular congregation. This view is expressed by Lucy: "if I am in any way instrumental in helping to keep our synagogue, at least at the strength it has, and I wish it were stronger. I wish we were more in numbers. I wish we were all not older people, in the main. If I, in my lifetime, live to see that it still remains, it doesn't fold, I feel there's a reward for that. The fact that we've kept the Orthodox alive in Millerville. . . . If anything I'm doing has helped, I'm glad." Others mentioned that a steady relationship with God and religious community was mutually beneficial to the survival of each: "my life is divided into good social areas and then good retreat areas." Durkheim's eloquent yet simple statement that the idea of society is the soul of religion is an apt encapsulation of the many social needs that were met in formal participation in religious organizations (Durkheim, 1965, p. 466).

ATTENDANCE, MEMBERSHIP, AND FINANCIAL SUPPORT

Among the older adults in the study, a fair number mentioned that there had been attenuation in some of the formal measures of participation in religion or of their religiosity. For a variety of reasons, regular attendance in formal worship had experienced the greatest degree of diminution, but as is evident from their engagement and involvement with daily prayer, these attenuated formal links may not be the most salient parts of religious experience among older adults. Moreover, attendance is perhaps not as indicative of commitment to faith or to a particular congregation when people are comparatively long-standing and for some, lifelong, members of a congregation. The relatively high level of stable community residence, stability in terms of employment, stability in marital relationships, and stability of membership in religious congregations, all combine to provide well-anchored social moorings for individuals. Changes in levels of formal participation in religion are amenable to adjustment, not elimination, because there is such a thick social context surrounding individuals as well as their continuing practice in the folkways of faith. Attendance as well as other formal religious activities are open to change without imperiling beliefs or folkways. When asked about attendance, Martha said it was important to "go, to listen to the service and the message the minister prepared for that Sunday. . . . I can see how after you get a certain age, it's still important but you just don't have the initiative to get ready and prepare yourself. Your body seems like it's drained, it has nothing to do with your not loving the Lord or the faith you carry, there's just something about your body that changes."

At minimum, community-dwelling elders were regular attendees at formal worship throughout the year and consistent participants in some activities related to their congregations. Many were lay leaders on committees over the course of many years of their lives, yet they did not see themselves as intensely religious or spiritual. This is not to say that people were always cognizant of this or discontented about their connection to religion. One person said her efforts in religion were directed toward "being a better person, being good. I'm no saint after all." In other words, formal participation in religion and faith, as well as financial support according to one's means, were a continuation of "doing what is expected."

Margaret, a long-term care resident, attends mass weekly when it is offered. "We don't even have to go out of the building. We just walk across, and they have church every week, and it's just wonderful. Mass every week. If not, they have a very lovely lady that puts on a very good [service]. I guess they're [priests] so busy today and shortage and so forth—then they'll have a prayer service. And that's about every other Sunday, whenever the priests are unavailable. Oh, it's lovely, yes. And so helpful. All we do is just go across into the building." Another long-term care resident, Douglas, notes that his participation was the main and almost only connection with faith at the same time that he admits that he "wouldn't put anything into" his participation. The pattern of regular churchgoing established in his youth was maintained throughout his adult life until his move to a nursing home. In this long-term care setting it is difficult to make arrangements for formal worship outside the facility. He describes his participation as "not much now . . . I'd go [back then], I felt that it was my duty to go to church, to go to mass. I wouldn't miss it. I was good that way. But I wouldn't put anything into it. I would have my envelope, put my envelope in. That would be it. That's it. Good-bye." He participates in other devotional activities offered regularly within the nursing home, but mass is not part of that and he does not particularly miss it.

Though I did not ask specific questions about financial support of their respective congregations currently or over a lifetime, many people offered their own comments about the kind of financial support they had provided to their congregations. Some also volunteered that their support had been forthcoming and reliably so, but that their families had to come first on many issues of money. Many, if not most of the older adults in the study, grew up in families where money was not available in generous amounts and though some had climbed the ladder of upward mobility to reach a point where finances were not a continuing source of worry and insecurity, others had not. Contributions to their congregations by some of the financially well-endowed were substantial, yet there were also many examples of the tale of the widow's mite; that is, people whose contributions were valuable because they provided as much financial support as they could offer and did so in a willing spirit. One example from Alice's life at two different points illustrates this point. "When we were married in Stanton, and the Three Saints Church was built upstairs [renovated], it was funny. We were married a couple years and we had two hundred dollars saved. So, we were the first ones in the parish to donate that two hundred dollars, for a small window on the right-hand side in the big church. And, in fact, our name is in there." "And then in Barrville, the St. Peter's Church, when they were getting new pews and everything, we donated some money. Enough for one pew and our name is on it. You have to look for it, you know? But, like I say, I never went looking for it. I figure it's there."

The strength of these long-term ties to the religious congregation and to the various groups that conduct a host of activities in support of the church locally and institutionally is seen in these remarks from Alice, who has been in a nursing home for two years. She mentioned spontaneously that " . . . I belonged to the Ladies' Guild and the Rosary Society. The other day I got a card from the Rosary Society. Yes, once a year they send it to you. I can't get up there like I used to. But they still remember me." It was important for many of the long-term care residents to be remembered by members of their former parishes. Long-term care residents realized that they were no longer an active part of the congregation, but they were aware and appreciative of small and large efforts made by the congregations and members to acknowledge and remember them. Their former congregations were important reference groups for long-term care residents, and some had periodic contact with people from their congregations during annual or semiannual outings or get-togethers. Three people had more frequent interaction with friends from former congregations for lunches, shopping trips, and other day trips for concerts, art exhibits, and similar social events.

CREATING NEW FOLKWAYS OF FAITH IN LATE LIFE

FOLKWAYS OF SERVICE: "GOD NEEDS A LITTLE HELP ONCE IN A WHILE, TOO"

Walter, 70, prays and reads the Bible regularly. He also attends formal worship weekly. Yet one of the ways that he has forged a new folkway of faith is through an act of ecumenical, religious service he fell into a few years ago. "Now I'm really going to shock you [laughs]. I got a phone call about three years ago from one of the women in [another residential tower], and she said, 'What are you doing tomorrow?' I said, 'Well, I haven't any special plans.' She said, 'Do you want to go to a funeral?' I said, 'You're sick.' I said, 'Why would I want to go to a funeral?' She said, 'Well, I belong to the Funeral Ministry of St. Simon's Cathedral, and we'd like to have eight people.' Now, what it is—there are eight people that come in, and we wear a red badge with a white cross on it, and we escort the body. We meet it at the door, and we escort it out, and we sit through the mass. . . . And this is done for elderly people who don't have any family left. We've had women—we had one woman who was a hundred and two years old. We've had funerals there where there wasn't one single soul in the church for this person's funeral. And it's just that I feel, 'Hey, you don't have to be a Catholic to wish somebody a safe journey to heaven,' so I do it. I've been doing it for three years."

Walter elaborates on his participation in the "Funeral Ministers" group by saying that "I thought I was doing something nice for that person. You know, I think it must be a terrible thing to die and not have anybody around you to see you off or anything. Of course, we all know that that person is not in that box. . . . The soul has gone, immediately upon death. But I end up doing three or four months in a row because they're always so short. And a cute little thing about this is that the woman that got me involved in this, I went down to Deer Park last week for the weekend, and I decided to stay a couple of extra days because the weather was so beautiful, and we went to the [a playhouse] to see a play. And I called her and told her that I wouldn't be back Monday to do the funeral, but it wasn't my turn anyway. And she said, 'Oh, I don't know what we're going to do. We're going to be short.' I was naming off the people in the group, and I got to her name and she said, 'Well, I can't make it.' And I said, 'What do you mean, you can't make it?' She said, 'Well, you know I bowl on Monday.' And I said, 'When did bowling come ahead of God?' And she got frustrated. I said, 'You know, Doris, you make commitments to a certain thing. You have to do it.' Of course, she thinks she's got to go bowling."

CREATIVE ENGAGEMENT LINKED TO FAITH BUT MOVING ALONG NEW PATHWAYS

Though virtually everyone in the study grew up into traditional folkways of faith, there were a few people whose activities had spilled over into creative and helpful forms of engagement that reinforced the person's core orientation but also moved them beyond the familiar patterns they preserved. An illustration of this is found in an ongoing activity recounted by Gwen. Though active in traditional religious arenas, Gwen started writing poetry while recovering from a significant stroke: "Most of it [the new activity] I did because in 1991 I had a stroke. And I think it was all because of feeling depressed and needing help; so I had to force myself to think good thoughts and bright and cheerful thoughts because I didn't want to sit back and make, pull other people down to feeling depressed because I did. So I try to make people want to be around me, and they're not going to want to be around me if I'm going to be sad and down. So I try to boost myself and in order to boost myself I try to boost them too."

Like the poetic scribes, Esteban and Manuel, in Thornton Wilder's *The Bridge of San Luis Rey*, Gwen often writes poems and short expressions of sentiments for others. People come to her and she talks with them about what they'd like to say. She then creates poems for them to use in a variety of ways. Gwen has published some of her own work in local newspapers, and we ended our interview with a discussion of the merits of contributing a poem to a national contest. This creative, new folkway does not supplant her continued participation in religious activities, but it permits her to grow and move beyond real physical limitations that she cannot alter. Gwen no longer attends formal worship services. Any direct participation with her congregation takes place in her own home, and though these occasional visits for Communion are not ones she wishes to abandon, she observes that it is not the same as "being in church." The poetry and writing bring people to her and are now a new way of putting religious belief and behavior into her life in a meaningful way. A friend of Gwen's calls her poetry "drawing with words."

New Folkways Within a Long-Term Care Setting

Carol, 79, has lived in White Pines for nearly a decade and has had serious, chronic health problems. Yet her description of faith and religious engagement also features new ways of "doing religion" in late life from her room in an institutional setting. "Oh, when I came here [nine years ago], as soon as I was able to do it, I did the mail every day. And on the weekend, well, on Saturday, I get a room roster, Roman Catholic, so that I go to each room and new people. I go to them, as well, and ask them you know, find out whether they're well enough to come to the service. Whether they would like to. If they are not able to come to the service, I bring the Eucharistic minister on Sunday, and we have the service at ten o'clock. And when the service is over, then we go around to all of the rooms and all the people. And last week, and this is about average, seventy-eight received. Some are not able to swallow. Then we say a prayer for them. But that's what I told them about at [a medical center], that I felt that, it may seem, it's a very small part of it, but it makes me feel if I'm bringing a person and the good Lord together. And even the prayer, if they're not able to receive, the good Lord knows that. So, I honestly think the good Lord left me around, maybe, to do those things. I no longer do the mail because I couldn't keep that up." Just before we close the interview she says this about how she sees herself. "My faith is very important. I think I'm a survivor of cancer, in a nursing home, and managing to do good."

For those in long-term care settings who do not have a sufficient level of health and stamina to get out to do reading programs or religious activities, the lack of opportunity to give God a little help is detrimental. This is poignantly evident in the following exchange with Sarah, formerly an active member of a congregation. "The synagogue. And I worked hard . . . I had good, good help. That's what it is. You can't do it alone. I had a good committee. But you've got to know how to do it right, to get them to do it. And though, sometimes I miss it . . . I miss feeling important."

BENDING AND NOT BENDING THE FOLKWAYS OF FAITH: ADAPTATION TO CHANGE

Two phrases emerged spontaneously in a number of interviews and were used separately to describe the degree of adaptation made in the individual's understanding and practice of faith. They were: "I have not bent my faith," and seemingly in the opposite vein, "I have bent a little in what I do." Another thought, captured in this phrase, "I have learned to bend in certain ways," was characteristic of a handful of responses. These expressions were offered in response to two concerns that were at odds with one another. For those who stated that "I have not bent my faith," the firm beliefs that they adhered to had not, they emphasized, "bent" over time and across the course of life. However, among this group were some who said that although their faith, i.e., beliefs, had not been bent, they had learned to accept major changes in the way that formal worship services were organized. The changes people had bent for included accepting the shift from Latin and other languages to English in the Catholic mass; embracing the inclusion of the laity within formal worship in ways that they had never considered or imagined would happen; and accommodating the new roles open to women and the increase in women filling roles in formal worship or in support of activities related to it. The steadfast beliefs basic to the particular denomination, and in most cases to the broader Christian and Jewish religious traditions, endured without much temporizing or qualification.

Notwithstanding this broadly based adherence to beliefs themselves, most had learned to change at least a small set of particular behaviors that had been as much a part of childhood socialization as the beliefs had been. An illustrative instance of this kind of change was identified

by Jewish women in the study. Though there have been increasing
numbers of older Jewish women in reform traditions, some of whom
are presently holding Bas Mitzvahs in late life because this ritual had
not been open to them as girls, no one in the study had held one for
herself. Some whose daughters were themselves among the young-old
or close to this age boundary had also missed the experience of the
Bas Mitzvah. Yet in the third generation of the granddaughters the
bending had occurred, Bas Mitzvahs had been held, and the change
was called "bending in the right direction." A truism about social change
is that as a process it unfolds slowly or lags and affects groups unevenly
even when the change itself is most dramatic. With respect to religious
behavior, as described by people in this sample, one sees perhaps just
how slow the pace is. Even those in the distal generations (third and
fourth generations from the person interviewed) do not have fresh
rituals. Folkways surrounding religion and faith are substantially intact,
even if a few have been tweaked a bit or "bent" at the edges. The system
of religious beliefs, the sacred ideology, if you will, is robust. And though
interactions and folkways of religion are slightly more amenable to
bending than beliefs are, the bending has been gradual and is now
part of a largely taken-for-granted acceptance of religious reality intact
among older adults.

The degree of disapproval for certain changes undertaken in the
folkways of faith among distal or third and fourth generations provides
a glimpse into the areas where older adults did not wish to bend or
see others bending. For example, elders were not successful at masking
their distaste for contemporary clothing and behavior they encountered
in formal, religious services among younger participants. The charitable
word, casual, was used to describe current fashion among the young
and this trend was almost universally disdained by elders. Some older
women did admit to wearing slacks to formal worship, and most of the
oldest members of the study had adjusted their schedule of formal
worship and participation in congregational committees, but the established folkways were woven into their individual practices almost seam-
lessly, so for most, bending was inconceivable. Those residing in long-
term care facilities did much more bending or adapting to the reality
of living in a controlled environment that placed other health and
organizational priorities at the top of how life was to unfold. Nonetheless, there were examples of bending folkways of faith. These instances
shed some light on what is amenable to modification and suggest some
of the contextual elements or occasions that stimulate the process of
bending folkways of faith.

BENDING AS ADAPTATION

Barbara was one of several people who had noticed and adapted to the more active roles that women currently played in religion. In her denomination, women are now represented among the clergy and she expresses the genuine astonishment, "I never thought I'd be alive when they ordained women," that others shared. Others had made accommodations earlier in life when they faced concrete dilemmas. For some, their own marriages had posed various social situations that required changes in thinking and behavior. For others, intermarriage or switching religious affiliation was part of their children's and grandchildren's lives; and was something they adapted to flexibly in late life in ways that they would have rejected as younger people. Anne discussed the quiet ways in which adaptations to childhood religious socialization began to occur for her as she made her own life as a young adult. "Yes, I had a great love [for religion]. I still love the mass to this very day. But in thinking back, I see there were things though. Catholicism and I were kind of a little bit out of tune, because you can see back then when mixed marriage was such a taboo, I still went ahead and did [it]. I still did not think that mixed marriage was wrong, as long as I kept my own faith and I didn't change his faith. Each of us kept our own, but it was absolutely unbelievable—the attitude. I was about to go to hell and I was in mortal sin and this and that and the other. And actually, it was through an assistant pastor's kindness and understanding, that he even gave me permission to marry, because my pastor said, 'I will never give you permission to marry.' "

Clara talks about the fact that many ideas and practices once promoted by her religion have changed. "At one time attending the Eastern States Exposition [New England's version of a state fair] was frowned upon," but "if you read your Bible, you know pretty well what to do and what not to do. You don't lie and steal and commit adultery and all that stuff [because you attend a fair]." Attending the exposition and other entertainment or being part of an array of social activities have had more latitude with Clara. As firm as her commitment to religion has been, she does act independently and in ways that bend conventional ways of doing religion. This is illustrated in the fact that she and her husband were married by a Salvation Army preacher. They passed up their own minister in a church where they were members for another minister whom they liked very much. Defining the situation, even a religious and sacred one, would seem to be as much of an interactional prerogative as it is a structural one. This may help explain how most of the Roman Catholics had adapted quickly to the many changes of practice and in the interpretation of church teachings. One example of a typical, unproblematic adaptation and bending to changes wrought by Vatican II and its cascade of openness is seen in remarks by Val, "It didn't bother me. In fact, I thought it was better because I understood more." She recounts the dramatic way that many practices changed, particularly in terms of what she had been taught as a child and young adult. In response to a question about women becoming priests, her answer contained the forthright, practical, and adaptive stance that was characteristic of others' perspectives. She replied, "I think it's going to come to that because there's a shortage. It wouldn't bother me. It's God's doing and people need religion no matter who it is [leading]."

BENDING IN TERMS OF THE VIEW OF CLERGY AND THEIR ROLES

This sample, as I have suggested, owes its deep commitment to belief and observance in large part due to its generational standing within a society and a period of history that featured religious affiliation and a moderate degree of involvement as an unquestioned part of the social order. People did what was expected and were taught religious beliefs and joined religions and carried their faith with them. Thus, it is not surprising to note that older adults offered some insight and commentary about their perspectives on the role of the clergy and the impact of clergy on the engagement with folkways of faith.

Some people in the study had what I like to call instant editors built into their understanding of clergy in their religious communities. This instant editor came into play like a toggle switch in that many people in the study turned off thoughts that had been flowing in one direction in order to comment on the clergy's role in their own religious development and over the years within a congregation. Many recognized that not every clergy member preached well or related well to members either individually or collectively (clergy were not permanent fixtures in their own religious communities, and among those who discussed a clergy role, there had been experiences with three or more members of the clergy within the same congregation). There were a few instances where the quality of relationships with clergy was a factor in moving people to membership by bringing them into a congregation, or by stimulating their movement to another congregation in the same de-

nomination or into a congregation that was further along the denominational continuum. Usually the moves to other congregations were, to
take a phrase from the parlance of professions and occupations, lateral
moves. In other words, some people described the role that clergy
played in creating turnover among members. In a different vein, others
described turnover in clergy as something they had to "live with" until
the time for another change in leadership. Two people described the
logistics of a phenomenon that they had not anticipated living through,
that is, the merger of their congregations with other congregations.
The merged congregations were spoken of as "settled" after initial
difficulties, but the joinery of the merger was characterized as weak.
Normal cycles or events faced by the religious community resulted in
greater than normal stresses. An example of this was provided by someone who was serving on a search committee for a new cleric. Among
the final candidates interviewed were three women, two of whom were
not married and one who had "switched" denominations some years
ago; one homosexual male; and two others whose educational backgrounds were not up to the level of either one of the formerly independent congregations now merged and in their first search for a religious
leader. It was a "new world" for them even when it came to hiring
a minister.

The issue of clerical leadership was not something I asked older
adults to consider, but for a few whose congregations were in the throes
of change, it was a topic on their minds and one that seemingly was
forcing them to reexamine some of their reliance on traditional or
customary responses. Social change in the pool of ministerial candidates
was compelling a couple of older members to face the larger realities
of where the congregation, and they as members, were headed. The
steadiness of religious involvement among the group of older adults
was likely influenced by the steadiness, even in a systematic rotation,
of the clerical leadership. In some congregations that dependable feature is itself endangered by external social forces. No one here had
been part of a congregation that had ceased to exist, but several people
from very different congregational settings were well aware of and mentioned explicitly the lack of younger members and the difficulty of
encouraging regular participation among younger people. There were
some other perspectives on the role of clergy that are worthy of mention here.

Clara, for example, was concerned about the purpose and role of
clergy with respect to salvation and members of the congregation.

"There's one thing that I don't agree with that goes on in my own church—I think the pastors should be studying the word and praying and learning to teach the people, rather than run the business end of the church. I think their deacons should run the business end of the church, and they don't do that today. . . . But that's very scriptural. . . . The pastor gets so involved with the business end of the church, that he doesn't bring—he doesn't feed the people the word like he should, I don't think. That's my opinion." This concern about the financial end of the clergy role and the perception that business was taking a lead in the attentions of clergy was shared by a few others in the study.

Clara's perspective as well as her own ability to define and redefine the situated commentaries and messages provided by clerics appears in Rose's remarks. Her comments about what she takes away from worship were framed within a role as a believer who actively interpreted religious content from the pulpit. The translator related Rose's perspective in this way, " . . . another thing she was saying about services was that she likes the preaching, but there are some preachers that—she doesn't like what they say, or she doesn't agree with what they say. But at the same time, she's saying that for sixteen years, she feels like she has the knowledge to take the good and get rid of the bad messages." This ability to use an instant editor to reframe or shift focus is a way to shape received information according to the recipient's understanding or definition of what message needs to be taken away.

BENDING IN TERMS OF CHANGING RELIGIOUS AFFILIATION

Another theme that captures some variation in the adaptive experiences articulated by older adults in the study is likewise found in Rose's comments. Rose had a major turning point in midlife when she was preparing for major surgery. A priest who came to the hospital insisted that she "make confession" if she wanted to receive Communion. She didn't believe in confession, and would not make confession, so she was not given Communion. This episode was very upsetting to her. After Rose returned home from successful surgery, an "aunt invited them [Rose and her husband] to go to [the aunt's] church and they did." This worship was a totally different experience for wife and husband. Once Rose started going there regularly, she "started reading the Bible and praying directly to God, and it's been sixteen years since that day," and Rose is still a conscientious member of a religious group that is a charismatic Catholic group. Rose spends part of the year in Millerville where her daughter and grand-daughter now live, and the other part of the year in the country of her birth. While in the United States, she attends Pentecostal services in a congregation close to her daughter's home. Services are in Spanish. She is happy with her change in affiliation and with both congregations. She says through the translator "that the happiness of being in the house of God . . . is like when you get married and you go to your parents' house, and you're happy and joyful to be with your parents. Well, it's the same experience when she goes to church."

Some people were also aware in very personal and concrete ways of the consequences of rigid orthodoxy and of the impulse toward fanaticism that makes some religions the only correct religions in the eyes of adherents. Most people in the study had to make some kind of adjustment to whatever residual concerns they might have had about the righteousness of their religion's worldview. Most often those residual concerns were evoked by family, usually adult children, or grandchildren, intermarrying, or in the changes that others close to them had experienced. Marilyn tells, for example, of attending Roman Catholic mass for most of her married life even though she did not officially convert from her own faith to Roman Catholicism until some years after her husband's death. Two others had confronted instances of adult children's membership in contemporary religious cults.

Other than two people whose beliefs, and occasionally, practices, brought them into roles that were very close to evangelization, older adults did not endorse wearing religion publicly so as to present oneself as possessing a kind of righteous authority. Many refused to criticize the sacred beliefs others held and practiced and did not endorse "pushing" their beliefs on others. In this context, the long-term care settings sometimes posed religious issues to residents. Specifically, three people interviewed from long-term care facilities observed that they had been subjected to regular encounters with visitors whose religious beliefs were not synonymous with their own. Two of the three used the word proselytize to describe these encounters. Talking with others is a valued social interaction, particularly in long-term care settings where individuals often had limited kinds of social interaction. Two people thought they had been approached as one human being to another, only to discover that there was a pointed conversation and purpose to the interaction. Since they did not desire to be converted religiously, they had to forgo the conversation and felt hoodwinked by the proselytizers. With one exception, a person who routinely sends donations of money to a televangelist, the older adults did not directly support proselytizing activities.

Though there was a lack of support for evangelization, it is the case that several people in this sample had changed their religious affiliations or had converted from one denomination to another. Most had converted while younger and for reasons generally associated with the transition to marriage and family roles. These instances and occasions were described in chapter 3. However, there was one instance of conversion that occurred during late life and another of conversion during late middle age. Both are worth noting in order to highlight similarities with other conversions and because they are exceptional in terms of patterns in the group as a whole.

Unlike Marilyn, who had converted some time after her husband's death, Anne married outside the church when young but had remained a loyal member for a good part of her life. When her marriage faltered, she had to face a lack of support and understanding of her dilemma and her family's difficulties from her own religion and its congregational community. She describes the process of change that unfolded. "I would always stay faithful to the Catholic Church. It took me a long time to get to the point to break. And then I realized, as time went along, I said, 'You know, I've given all my heart and my love and devotion to this church, but the times I've needed you most is the time you give me pain. You give me problems on top of my problems.' So little by little then I started going to all these other churches . . . I was out. I went to Unitarian. I went to Methodist. I went to—I was searching."

"I would still be going to mass. I never stopped going to mass for some strange reason. I'm still going to mass today but it's a different feeling when I go to mass, okay. I'm going to mass in a different way than I went before. I still love the mass and whatever; that's not the problem. The problem is that I, in thinking back, I did not really belong, you know, as a Catholic, according to the way they want a Catholic to function, because I wasn't functioning as your typical Catholic. . . . I was saying, 'Look, I'm giving you all the love and devotion I have.' And I'm finding all, I'm finding that . . . I'm not getting the response back that I think I need. And a lot of other Catholics have felt the same way. And then when I saw that paperwork involved, as far as annulment. And there was this wonderful lady that I met in the Unitarian church in [another state]. I'm telling you, she exemplified everything that the

Catholic Church is always preaching, and she is a Unitarian. . . . I even went to the Jewish temple in [that same state]. At that time they were battling between the Reform and the Orthodox. And I was received so well and so hospitably that they even asked me to sit in on the choir. . . . This is what I think God is all about. And then years later, . . . I'm hearing Father say from the altar, 'Let's wish our Jewish friends happy holidays.' And I'm thinking, 'God, after all these years, you're finally wishing your Jewish friends happy holidays. Thank God for that. You're making a step after all those years.' And then we finally hear the pope apologizing for all the sins of the Catholic Church.

"And I finally went into the Episcopal Church one day. And then I thought my God, the prayers were exactly the same; everything's the same. I mean, I could just, you know, pick up," which is what she did. Today Anne also meditates and reads a variety of literature that reinforces aspects of religious and spiritual beliefs that her formal participation does not as a rule provide. She had been living in a long-term setting for 1 year at the time of our interview, and she is the atypical person in the sample as a whole with respect to her ongoing "search" for the right fit between religion and herself. "You need a home base to let you kind of be a free spirit . . . it's like when a child outgrows the parents, I guess. You know, the shoe starts pinching but you still go back to the factory for a pair of shoes. [chuckles] No, I didn't go back, but I've been going to school on my own ever since . . . I mean, when you start exploring is when you find these wonderful answers to things that there are no answers for sometime until you search a little bit. And you do meet wonderful people. So I'm still learning. I think if there was one room in the house or one room in this world and they say, 'Which room would you choose out of all the rooms?' I would say the library. Because if you do well in the library you're going to do well everywhere else. If you can read and learn, you'll survive."

She sums it up. "I think I'm in a better place now for going through what I went through. I think if I hadn't been uncomfortable, I think I'm in a better place now for . . . searching. I would have missed all those wonderful things that I found. So I think along with that awful pain I was going through, the way I was resolving my pain also led me to other things, that if I had been totally happy in my little corner I never would have found. . . . I would have been in my little group and I never would have ventured out of the little parish boundaries. And that would have been it. I would have been set there, okay, which maybe would have been fine for somebody. But I wouldn't, I don't think I, it wouldn't be me and I wouldn't have found what I did find. So that's why it's kind of hard for me to be, to go back and revert to the thinking of someone who never left their little parish, you know. . . . But the thing is we have to realize that when I start thinking back, my mother left her home at what? 15. She was married at 16 in America. She left her parents and whatever. Then what I did is I migrated. I left [the religion], it's part of the life process, that's all, you know."

"I'M NOT A FANATIC, BUT . . . ": A DISCLAIMER WITH RESPECT TO RELIGIOUS IDENTITY

Some older people in the study realized that they could very well have been born into social situations with other, very different, religious beliefs. Thus, with only two exceptions, there was a clear and pronounced view that with regard to previous and present religious affiliation or identity, this specific identity was not the only way to be connected to the divine or to God. Some elders had acquired knowledge about other ways of thinking about the sacred through courses offered in their local communities through senior centers, educational institutions, and in one case, through a congregation's educational programming. Given the localism and stability of residency in this sample, this kind of general awareness, of the many ways to God, speaks of a willingness to be open and to learn about other religions and ways of relating to the transcendent. Indeed, many older adults, including those in the long-term care sample, expressly stated that they were not "fanatics" about forcing their beliefs on others or about following through with their own faith's folkways. Statements abounded such as: "I'm not a fanatic, but I have to have St. Theresa's statue nearby." "I'm not a fanatic, but I make a point to attend [a formal prayer group] every week." The prevalence of this disclaimer (Hewitt & Stokes, 1975) in the comments of older adults was notable and constitutes an unstated awareness that others may regard the behaviors identified as indicative of an overcommitment to religion. Disclaimers are preliminary phrases used by people to preserve the identities they present at the same time that they wish to distance themselves in some fashion from negative connotations that members of a culture or society typically attach to that identity. With respect to religious belief and behavior, older adults widely used a disclaimer that was generally phrased this way: "I'm not a fanatic, you know, but I am religious." The use of the word fanatic was itself interesting in that it was not attached to a specific religious group or denomination and seemed to reflect a more general image of any person whose religious ideas and behavior exceeded normative boundaries; that is, someone who "overdid" religion. Often there was an implicit distinction drawn between "fanatics" and "saints." It is important to mention that these two terms were not used to describe the same kind of behavior or thinking. In other words, there was no attempt to join these words in an oxymoron or as a useful way to make a point.

Donna voiced a refrain found in the words of many others in the study. She said that while religion is "there," that is, in her life as a real and meaningful aspect, she was not "over-religious. I'm like half-and-half." Pauline considers herself a religious person but does not "go around boasting and looking down on people that aren't." "You don't have to be religious to be good, you can be good without being, I am not a fanatic, you know." Gwen says she is religious but, "Not overly. Just . . . because like I don't like to be overbearing. But only God and I know how much I am religious, that's how I am. I like to believe my way, and as deep as I believe, and that is between the person and God. I don't believe in idols. I don't—I mean, I'm not praying to a tree—I know God." One long-term care resident, Douglas, put it this way, "I believe in religion. But to me religion's a private matter. It's a very private matter. To a point where you just don't advertise it. You don't broadcast your feelings. I don't mind blessing myself in front of [people], you know. I'm not ashamed. But there's no need of going out and preaching it like, that's what turned me off a lot to this is these preachers, these television evangelists, certain ones. And the ones that try to put the pressure on you." Maxine was reluctant to describe herself as spiritual or religious: "I probably wouldn't want to [use] the word 'religious'; it means different things to different people. And I do not think that that pertains to me. Better to say, if it's possible, that I'm living as I think the Lord would want me to live. And this is heading toward the inevitable, when the day of reckoning arrives. That's the only thing that I'm concerned with. Not with people's judgment, but with the Lord's judgment."

AWARENESS AND MEANING OF RELIGIO-ETHNIC DIFFERENCES

Some elders, particularly those who were black or Jewish, but a few others as well, namely Irish Catholics, were keenly aware of the problems of belonging to a non-mainstream religion in a society that values freedom of religion and equality. The relationship between certain kinds of religiosity and anti-Semitism and racism is well-documented in social scientific research. It is one of the many fascinating paradoxes about the effects of religious belief and behavior upon adherents. This was crystal clear in the comments of elderly Jews but was not restricted to or exclusively captured by them. Some of the Christians were sensitized to the walls that religious fervor had built in their lives. World War II and the Holocaust were referred to by many as the most telling example of religious and ethnic intolerance. A few added some current examples from the conflict in Bosnia and in some African countries. Among African-Americans, and as was the case with Jews, there was a deep-seated, general awareness that how others perceived them was inevitably connected to being different in ways like religion and ethnic background. In the instance of Jews and blacks, the religio-ethnic ascribed status was often not an issue personally, but was always a factor that had to be acknowledged and reckoned with socially and sometimes in their own congregations as well as across religions. The variation that existed among the perceptions of difference was in the strength or intensity of its impact on biographic identity shaped during early and young adult years of socialization. Pauline describes it this way: "We came to Connecticut, Laurelford—we were going to—there weren't any colored churches in Laurelford. I'm not the type of person that I have to go to a colored church or this or that. I'll go to any church. It doesn't matter, okay. But my sister wanted to belong to a [colored church]. Anyway, there was no . . . colored church, for all colored people here, so we started going to church in Samuelson. That was my uncle's church. We went there for twenty-two years. And, for some reason, it got burned down." After the destruction of that church, she and her family joined a church in a neighboring town much closer to their home in Laurelford than the Samuelson congregation had been. Many years later, when Pauline was 60, she changed membership again, becoming a member of a church in Laurelford—the same community that she calls home. Her understanding of the role played by color then and now is one that five of the six African-Americans noted when they discussed their religious membership and participation. Though most now belonged to integrated churches, some had attended all-black churches at various points in their lives, usually as children and adolescents, but not exclusively or only as younger people. The awareness of being different was something that both blacks and Jews in the study acknowledged and for themselves at least, they had arrived at some understanding that was a workable, balanced perspective that they were able to adopt during their discussion. For some this did not seem to be a wholly satisfactory stance, particularly given the prejudice and discrimination they had seen during their lives and that for some was a muted but present force today, but it was a broad, intellectual understanding that accounted for inequitable experiences without giving in to a gnawing resentment. It was a wise view of the deep reality that despite words to the contrary, not all were welcome as full participants in social institutions and that individuals had to make adjustments to that structure and change that structure when and if they had opportunity to do that. The effects of inequity are complex and complicated, particularly on the individual level of lives lived, but the biographical details reveal both the subtle and the gross role that being different plays in life, even in religious life, where soul and spirit are often thought to be unfettered by social considerations.

GENDER

Other than the starkly obvious and expected differences in the roles men and women were allocated and encouraged to assume to participate in their faiths and in society, there is scant evidence in these interviews of a gendered orientation to sacred beliefs and the accompanying behaviors or folkways of faith. Men and women were active and served in different ways within their congregations, but there was no strong or clear evidence that prayer, the most important folkway of faith, varied by being female or male. This muted gender effect was mildly surprising. Yet if residential stability and the bedrock early socialization to religion and faith are of the import I contend they are among this group, the lack of gender variation is consistent with what one might expect in this sample of pre-World War II generations. Women were gratified to see changes in how liturgical and other roles (pastoral ministry) were opening to them and to their children and grandchildren, but men in the study were equally receptive to these changes. Men were not vehemently or even mildly opposed to the changes. Perhaps the openings for women are coming at a time when the diminished status of religion makes any change acceptable or tolerable to people because the change permits continued survival of faiths in an increasingly secular social world in the U.S. Or perhaps they have acquired some age-related or experiential insight into gender inequity and to the opening up of religious roles that has occurred within their later years. The reason for their open acceptance of women in a variety of religious roles is unclear, but it is apparent that they are receptive to this large change.

Where gender mattered and showed itself clearly was in the dual tracks that pervade most religions and congregations; namely with respect to the formal leadership, clerical and lay, in the hands of men and the service and support activities with the women. This is such a pervasive part of the context that it contrasts with otherwise significant changes in women's roles as clergy and lay associates within various religions. Although a few people commented on this, most underlined that there was more than enough work to go around in the congregation and it appeared that for men and women there were more than sufficient opportunities to participate in highly valued and status-enhancing social and congregational activities. In other words, neither women nor men commented about gender inequity in local or congregational religious activities even though both men and women referred in positive terms to the larger changes evident in the religion and the congregation for women.

THE RAINBOW ESCAPING: NATURE AND THE DIVINE

Nature and things related to nature; not environment, not ecological concern, but deep appreciation and engagement in everyday aspects of the natural world in which all life unfolds, from gardening to observing backyard wildlife, to caring for pets and being attuned to cycles of nature were mentioned frequently as a noninstitutional domain of religiosity for older adults. Often this understanding was a kind of parallel track to the divine and complemented institutional forms of religion, but there were one or two people who had gradually come to the realization that for them, being in a natural setting (and preferences for natural setting varied) was just as important as participating in formal or structured collective observances.

Eugene sees religion and faith as private and reflective as well as communal and public: "Sometimes you feel like talking to the Lord, when you're out tending the garden, and no one is around to bother you." He does this and finds it a different way of connecting with what is otherwise a larger and more routine experience of going to mass and praying privately with standard prayers. It is a seasonal and occasional, but perhaps deeper sense of connection with what is divine.

Robert told a story that defined something about his characteristic orientation to life as well as to the natural world. He had worked in a jewelry store after retiring from the full-time work he pursued most his life. He loved the precious and semiprecious stones that were the stock in trade, and tells a wonderful story about the opal. "People would come in and I would say they were, perhaps, middle-aged or so, and I could see that they were people that I could tell this little story to. I would talk about opal, explain the different colors and so on, and this was the story that I would tell them. . . . I said that the good Lord created angels to see how man lived, how he behaved, how he loved nature and such. And one of these days, the angels saw the rainbow for the first time. And knowing how man abuses beauty, nature-wise and all, they cut a piece of the rainbow and buried it. Now, every time an opal is mined, that's part of the rainbow escaping [laughs]."

Robert walks daily. These walks are living examples of the overlap that some members of the study associated with the natural world and their faith. He puts it this way, "I'm blessed. And that walk I do—it's my quiet time in a religious state." Yet he also takes time on this medita-tive daily walk to share a nod and a wave with others he may pass. "I'm happy when I start my day, so maybe a little wave like that will let an individual start their day in a happy mood." With his way of relating to the natural world and religion in mind, it is not a giant leap to under-stand that when Robert visits his wife's gravesite it's "not for grieving. I'll say, 'Good morning' to her, but then I do meditation and the quiet times there. And that's my time [of prayer]."

Others, like Anne and Julia, convey a reverence for the natural world and described natural settings as places where God can be found. Anne "loved outdoors and nature. It was something that perhaps fairly early on made me pause from activity to thinking about being more deeply thoughtful and feeling more deeply. And it was usually a solitary experi-ence. I did write some poetry as a result of this. . . . And the beautiful part of it is we're always—no matter how old we are and how far we are removed from our childhood, we're surrounded by it [nature]." Since her move into a long-term care facility, it has been more challeng-ing to find natural settings for reflection and prayer, so she walks in the vicinity of the facility in order to find such places and has been successful in finding some spots that she uses for prayer as the weather and her health permit. Julia is also inclined to seek out natural settings for contemplation and prayer. "Well, for instance, down in Shell Haven [in a southern state]. We live near a Catholic church down there. In the back of the church I discovered—I used to walk my dog there every day—they had this beautiful memorial garden, and there's a pond back there, and there's the Virgin Mary with the waterfalls, and nobody ever goes there! And so, to this day, when I'm down there—and a friend is sick, or I'm going to take a plane trip, or I'm afraid of something—that's where I go. It's not inside a church . . . I meditate. You know, I'll say a little prayer. Like, for instance, when I was studying for my comprehensive exams before I got [master's degree] I spent a lot of time over there. I used to take—because nobody was over there—I used to take my books and study. But it gave me this peaceful feeling. A feeling of peace. Yes. Like if I go down by our brook, there's just something about being by the water that I think is very spiritual."

Andrew found this connection to nature and God in a creative activity, woodworking, he still pursues at age 92. He demonstrates what he means by showing me pieces of wood—one that will be turned into a finished piece that he holds out for me to see. "We have two round pieces. But to put a piece of ordinary wood and start turning, as we call it—to watch that rough piece of wood turn out to something that comes to be a thing like that [a finished, turned table leg], is what I get the biggest charge out of. . . . It's a faith. Yes. It's a faith. It's a recognition of beauty in some sorts that comes with seeing a beauty of that kind. I don't mean to brag when I say that I think some of those things—some of those shapes—are beautiful [as they were originally and as they were "turned" or transformed into objects]." Others had comments similar to those expressed by Clara, comments that drew on their rural, agricultural roots where part of faith and belief in God was reflected in the appreciation for the land and for the experience of working the land. "Well, yes. It has to be, don't it? Because when you're farming, you plow up the ground, sow the seed. You have to have faith that it's going to grow, don't you? Or you wouldn't put it in there. . . . You put that seed in there, you don't know if it's going to grow or not." Another artistic reminder of the free use and admixture of symbols and images from nature and religion is found in Lucy's home. In her kitchen there is a beautiful print, a circular contemporary representation of a garden, perhaps including a Torah. The inscription reads: "A person's good deeds are used by the one above as seeds for planting trees in the Garden of Eden. Thus, each of us creates our own paradise." The print, clearly displayed, evokes the quiet presence of the natural world in close kinship with a compatible religious ethos and underlines the strength of an association between the sacred and the natural world that was important to some people.

MYSTICAL EXPERIENCES

With respect to having sensed or felt a sacred or divine presence; that is, the direct experience or the presence of God at some point in their lives, the majority of older adults had not had mystical experiences. Most simply said they had never experienced God's presence and a few offered partial explanations. Larry says, "I suppose He's there all the time, but I never see Him. That's what we're taught, that he's there all the time, but you never see him." Andrew shares his puzzlement about this. "I can tell you that, no, I never have. And I wonder why. It seems to me that when a person is really, feels inside the love of God, that they have passed maybe through period of something when that has really shown up to them. They all of a sudden have developed that feeling of real faith, and that feeling has never happened to me. I have never had a feeling to come over me. No. I've never had that feeling. And I just don't know why, but I just can't get it."

Those few who spoke of a mystically felt presence described it as a physical experience of God being with them as they went about their daily activities and lives. This felt presence is distinguished from reports of out-of-body or near-death mystical experiences that have been documented in other research. Martha, for example, has not experienced God's presence in her own life, but she has some sense of what mystical experiences might be about albeit vicariously. She recounts her husband's talks with God during some parts of his final illness. There were many times when Ben told her that he had experienced God talking with him. Ben was called by name and God was beside him for a short while as they talked about present life. Martha thought it was likely that God could manifest a divine presence in this way, particularly to those like her husband who had great faith and had practiced that faith throughout life. For herself such a presence had not been felt. Another person had felt "the hand of God on my shoulder" once. These two instances are contrasted with the personal presence of the divine felt by Clara in the context of an ordinary day, "Oh, I've felt the presence of God many times. . . . Sometimes I've sat down here and I start to eat my breakfast and I ask the Lord to bless it. And I just actually feel the presence of God. Sometimes I just stop and thank him because I do feel his presence because he's with me. I can't even pray. I just have to thank him for his presence." Another example of a general, divine presence, but only for one time, is given by Maxine. "This was when my mother was living here. She was with me for eleven years. She was visiting a neighbor and I was sitting in the living room, by myself. Nothing was on, no radio, no TV. Nothing. The only sounds were the sounds of the birds singing. Doors were open. It was a beautiful day. And I felt a presence. It was just there. And I can remember that I was smiling and it just felt so peaceful and so good. And then gradually, it just kind of went away, and that was it. But it was real. It was real."

CONCLUSION

The patterns of religious behavior found among this group of older adults emphasize their continuous engagement with well-established folkways of faith. The most significant folkway identified by people was daily prayer. Prayers took several forms and exhibited some variation in content, though most prayer did not reach the level of reflection and contemplation. Martha's statement that "religion is something you carry with you," is both an apt and an accurate generalization about this group of older adults. Patterns of religious involvement with respect to prayer and to public participation in formal religious organizations and activities were carried by people into the stage of late life. It cannot be said of this group as Augustine once said about himself, "I have learnt to love you late" (Saint Augustine, 1961, p. 231). As we have seen in chapter 4 and here in chapter 5, the prevailing pattern of religious engagement is a steady one punctuated by some individual and collective adaptations or "bending" in particular ways of "doing" faith. Margaret Mead once said in writing about her early years that "I enjoyed prayer. I enjoyed church. I worried over the small size of our congregation" (Mead, 1975, p. 81). The elders in this study continue to enjoy these same folkways of faith and to worry about their respective congregations. They keep their faith and find it still among the most important ways of shaping their daily interaction, but even more, their orientation or perspective on life. As Sally concludes for herself and her husband, "The thing of it is, we were brought up, and his mother was very religious, we were brought up [this way]—we can't just walk away from it. That's it."

CHAPTER FIVE

A Grown-Up Faith With Musings, Doubts, and Questions

"I honestly don't know what I take away from the experience any more."

T hough there are theories and studies, chief among these Fowler's work (1981), that credibly posit and explicate a developmental model of faith development, such stages to faith development were not distilled from or evident in the interviews, particularly in the retrospective accounts, that emerged from this study. The underpinning of faith among these older adults was solidly built during youth and was maintained throughout life. There were adaptations to institutional and social change, which were for the most part gradually understood to be appropriate modifications of religion and were ultimately viewed as not disjuncture but a new way of doing things within the realm of the sacred. Consequently most older adults were connected to congregations and to their faith as a whole simply because faith remained a wellspring of meaning for their situated and biographic identities. Across the range of affiliations here (Catholic, Jew, Protestant) the pattern of keeping the faith in a fairly continuous pattern first established in childhood, does not speak to some of the departures from these sustained folkways of faith. Chapter 5 addresses some of the areas where participants in the study moved away from the seamless incorporation of religious beliefs and tenets. These doubts, musings, and questions were articulated by a small number of people, but they disclose some of the subtle variations in meaning that mark changes in what one once believed as a younger person to what one now believes or thinks about as an older adult. This discernible but quiet reflection is indicative of some movement away from mere acquiescence to tradition. Even among the steadfast and the sturdy there are inchoate reflections about beliefs, but such reflectiveness is not widespread. In this study, older adults found personal meaning and defined themselves with reference to a rather select set of folkways from their respective religions. Above and beyond subscribing to denominationally-framed and theologically based beliefs (many of which were not objects of intense reflection or personal scrutiny) and in participating regularly in local religious institutions through local membership and fairly regular participation, there was a strong sense of continuity. As an elderly woman (Deland, 1911, p. 246) stated early in the twentieth century, our later lives are linked to earlier times and realities. There is a bedrock grounding the range of choices we have. In her late life autobiography, Deland says, "I have said that we should decide whether we should rust out or wear out, but perhaps that was decided for us in our youth and in our middle age, for we are continually deciding all our life long what kind of old people we are to be. Every moment of our lives we are preparing for age; carving out the faces that we are to wear; moulding and modeling and casting our characters for good or bad." This chapter presents some of the areas where older adults offered thoughts about the ways in which they found in faith a continued source of identity, but one they had also redefined as a consequence of their experiences and of their understanding of how religion itself had changed over the years. Their thoughts contain musings, doubts, and questions that illustrate the capacity of individuals to decide how and what to take away from faith even in late life.

Beliefs about the divine have been significant social sources of meaning for believers and nonbelievers alike across history and across cultures. Though social scientific studies of religion as a meaningful basis for construction of self and identity have largely been consigned to side areas within respective disciplines, the value of understanding the ways in which individuals are influenced by religion has been at the heart of most social scientific research. Among the older adults interviewed in this study, religion and faith are important dimensions to the lives they have led and to the lives they now lead. The meaning of religion and faith is salient for some in the sense that beliefs about religion and faith shape their interactions with others and the ways in which they spend their lives. As Jean, a person whose life was shaped by formal and informal interactions related to faith, commented, "It's very important. I think without it I'd be kind of lost. Nowhere to turn. I think it helps a great deal to have religion. I've always been happy I've had it in my life." This sense of what sociologists call theodicy, the ability, or some would say function of religions to provide a way to understand the meaning of the ups and downs of living for their adherents, is echoed in the remarks of many elders in the study. Gwen, a Roman Catholic, can no longer attend weekly mass and now receives Communion in her home from members of her parish. These pastoral ministers come to her home once a week. She says she would deeply miss her participation if the pastoral ministers didn't come weekly. "Yes, because to me, like I always say, if I didn't believe in God I'd have nothing. You have to have something. You have to feel like you're a part of something and God made us. Who better to have something to belong to? . . . To me, I'd actually be afraid not to believe." Others commented on some of the traditional, theologically based beliefs of their respective religions: 96-year-old Sarah says that religion "gives you the hope and belief and faith, and belief in the hereafter. I believe there is a hereafter—Another life. Maybe another chance." Others like Ellen, 90, said, "I know, I know there is a God because I've seen him work to help me. I know. So if that's religion, of course, I don't take too much to organized religion." When she was interviewed, her beliefs and faith were working overtime to help her move through a serious health crisis that had placed her in an acute care setting within a long-term care facility. Her religious beliefs are "just holding me up because it seems—everything's getting worse. It seems like it is. But it's in his hands. I can't question it. But everyone says I look great. But some parts of me are all right but there's an awful lot that isn't."

Others like Andrew and Lydia were in advanced age more profoundly attached to tenets and practice of faith to such an extent that faith had come to define a larger outlook on themselves and others. In answering a question about what faith means, Andrew states, "Well, . . . what we have here, we have lived—I'm over 90, and Lydia is on the border of being 90—we have lived all these years—I say 64 years—I think we're 64 years married, and we have had a wonderful married life. We brought up our children and we're proud of all three of our children. We have really been blessed in many ways. And my feeling is that each Sunday that we go to church, I think of that as real blessings. Personally, I thank the Lord every day for the blessings that we have—every day we continue to enjoy our blessings. And church just magnifies that, as well as assuring us that as days go along . . . I feel assured that every day is going to be a good day." Lydia adds: "We live by faith. Without faith, it's impossible to please God. Because we have to have faith to even believe he exists. And if we believe he exists, then he makes himself known many times to us that it is not in a literal way, but spiritually; he reveals himself to us so that we know he's there." Their involvement with faith provides an assurance of hope in the present and of a future. It is not a trivial thing to carry faith and belief with one throughout life, and though it may appear to be a veneer that has endured for some it has been ingrained in identity. It is the frame for making sense of life and it provides hope about prospective turns in individual and social life. Perhaps this is the kind of hope that Kierkegaard envisioned when he said, " . . . certainly the eternal has range enough for the whole of life; therefore there is and shall be hope until the end. Therefore no particular age is the age of hope, but the whole of a man's life shall be the time of hope!" Kierkegaard expressly links hope to the "possibility of the good," and argues that "everyone who lives without possibility is in despair; he breaks with the eternal; he arbitrarily closes off possibility, and without the assent of eternity makes an end where the end is not" (Kierkegaard, 1962, p. 236). In their various religious traditions and current practices, most elders, no matter how much surrounded by pain and suffering, had not surrendered hope in the "possibility of the good." Faith in some dimension of the eternal provided by their religion or religious beliefs fostered the substance of that hope.

Where religious meaning had been stripped of its substance over the course of a person's life, the tone and implications of the person's observations are unambiguously resigned if not despairing. Larry's recent experiences are illustrative of this. Commenting on the meaning derived from his religion and faith, a person who had had lifelong participation in an array of roles, he said that now he does not find much meaning in belonging to his faith or congregation. He doesn't take much away from his faith. "And it's strange to me why it hasn't [given me anything]. We've been especially friendly with the ministers. But it didn't bother me when we didn't go to church this summer. And it wouldn't bother me if we didn't go this Sunday. I find it hard to find what there is in me that wants me to go when I really can't honestly say I get much out of it."

Many people literally used the expression, keep the faith, in various kinds of conversation. Julia observed that she uses this phrase occasionally and did most recently in an e-mail to friends, "And I ended up—keep the faith. Well, I think it means don't give up hope, keep trying, hang in there, you know? It means all those things to me." As to what faith itself is, definitions were fairly general but most embodied ideas that faith gave a larger perspective to the person's life and provided reassurance about having a purpose to one's life and to living. As Maxine says, "Faith comes in a lot of forms, I think. And it has developed because of living thoughtfully all these many years. And also, messages that I have been given over the years, from somewhere. They are there. As in the days after the death of my husband, it was made very clear to me that I must not—the mourning is a natural and normal thing—but I must not immerse myself in that too much, but think more about the thankfulness that I must feel in having had them for the years that they were here. And it was so clear, that I really have tried to live by that since then." When asked if faith gave her strength she says "Oh, absolutely. It's more than that. I think I'd rather call it support because we know on whom to lean. Yes. Support. I prefer that word." As she reflects about this she surmises that her definition of religion and faith " . . . might go back to a time when—a long time before [the present minister] was here. We had Bible Study classes we went to in the evening. The question was posed, 'Who is God?' And we were all given a certain amount of time to write down our feelings about what our response would be. And it just came extremely clear to me that there was only one—for me, anyway—there was only one word, and I just wrote down, 'God is love.' And there was nothing else. And . . . everybody else had much longer explanations, which was [sic] satisfying to them. You see, faith and God are such individual things, that they can be different things to different people. To me, God is love. God is when a child comes up and wraps his or her arms around your legs. That's God. Or the beauty of nature—whatever. Whether it be a snowstorm or a clear, blue sky. And faith must have a simpler explanation than long, verbose description. It lessens it, I think, when we try to explain it. It is something that is there like love."

QUESTIONS ABOUT LIFE AFTER DEATH

Questioning and wondering about major tenets of faith are signs of reflection, an intellectual and spiritual engagement with the typically unquestioned acceptance of religious beliefs and explanations (theodicy) that was characteristic of elders in the study. People with high levels of commitment and involvement in their religions were open about some of the areas that occasionally gave them pause. Sometimes people were concerned that I might misunderstand these doubts as perhaps indicative of greater misgivings, and their comments, were I think, adumbrated, in part as a way not to be misunderstood and in part because extending their remarks might actually lead to opening up some larger areas that would not withstand closer scrutiny. An instance of this is seen in Nora's response, "I don't remember questioning, except when somebody would die. Then my heart would break for them—I'd say, 'Why, God, did you take her?' Then I always felt that there was a reason for it, and I would become doubtful then. But maybe for that instant, I'd say, 'Why?' Then I'd say, 'Now I must try and understand he had a reason for this.' But that would be just for an instant, and then it was gone—any questioning." To dwell in this area, to challenge what is understood to be some part of a divine plan and a major tenet of a specific faith would be crossing into territory that the person was not ready or willing to explore. Yet there are doubts and questions for some and in the main those musings are largely unresolved or without definitive answers. This also speaks to a major flaw within most religions; namely, their inability to teach or expound upon their own principles to adults and adults in late life. It's not so much that ideas about God are misunderstood or that people needed or requested more information about the tenets of their faiths, but there was a perception among some that spiritual and religious education had been missing. This was most clearly found in the statements from Roman Catholics that the answers from the Baltimore Catechism did not stand as persuasive even for those who are the most committed and in-volved adherents.

In different words, this perspective is echoed in the words of one elder. "I'd like to say, 'Oh, you go to heaven.' There is no such a thing—I don't think so. Because nobody came back to tell us that there is. . . . Or, if I die, I'm going to go and see my mother and my father . . . no such a thing, either. You die, you go back to where you were born, made out of clay, sand, and you're going back to the same thing. Your body gets eaten up and the stuff that's left over is dirt. There isn't much left over." Another perspective comes from Arthur, a longtime former member of a synagogue who differentiates a core set of beliefs from other human constructions. "I believe—you see, the important thing, for me, is to believe in our Creator, and believe in the Ten Commandments. Those are the most important. But what was written after—I don't believe in that." Later this point is reiterated, "I believe in the Jewish religion, yes. But, like I told you before, I believe in our Creator with all my heart and soul. And I believe in the Ten Commandments. But whatever is written, it doesn't make sense to me. Take, for instance, food that comes from the sea—how can they say that it is not kosher? I cannot believe that!" Others had come to their own understandings as well. Walter, for example, did not believe in hell; God, yes, but not a place or an abstraction like hell. "I don't believe in hell. I don't believe in hell at all. I believe we make our hell on earth, and that we all go to the same place [after death]."

Others who had experienced untimely or unexpected deaths of loved ones had resolved many of the doubts they once had. Maxine expressed this best, though others had mentioned reaching similar understandings and one might say wisdom. Her losses help her to discuss death and sorrow with others. "I know what it is. And I think that that helps people to know that I'm telling the truth. Not just being casual about it. I really do understand. And another thing which was made very clear to me after the deaths, we must never say, 'Why me?' when things happen. And I have heard that from people. 'Why me?' 'Why me?' We have to remember that there is only one person on earth who can afford to say, 'Why me?' One perfect person. And he didn't, did he? He said, 'Thy will be done.' There was one particular case, and I really had to be a little bit tough on one person who was in this mode, and I said, 'Why not you? We are not exempt from anything. We are not promised anything. You can look through the whole Bible. We are not promised anything in that vein that we are going to go through life without pain, without something which is upsetting.' "

Wanda's musings about life after death lead her close to discarding or setting aside central religious beliefs. "Well, I, I don't know. Sometimes my aunt was like that and I know of others who were that way [abandoning a belief in God]. As we get older, you think more about death because you know you're not going to be around too many years. And you think about that a lot. And I do. I do. I think about that a lot. . . . I think there's a God but I don't know as I believe everything. That's awful to say."

Others with a belief in God also held some reservations about aspects of their religion's teachings. "I doubt hell a little bit. . . . Well, God is good. We believe that God is good. He's great. He's merciful. He's forgiving. He's this; he's that. Why would he torture people after they're dead? To hell? To burn in hell, which is scary. Why would he do that to someone unless they were, I really don't know what you'd have to do in order to go to hell, really. You know, you take a guy like Hitler.

But if he said before he committed suicide, 'I'm sorry, Lord,' he probably didn't go to hell. Who knows? . . . So I don't know, I've got a feeling that we're all going to the Promised Land of some sort."

DIFFERENT UNDERSTANDINGS OF WHAT LIFE MEANS

Pauline expresses tremendous sadness about the deaths of two of her daughters the year before the interview. For her part of faith is not just belief about life after death but "everybody don't feel the same about life. To me, life is important." She then tells how the second daughter who died "just about gave up" after her sister's death. This disturbs Pauline very much. "I get teary and emotional and it's not good, because she had everything in the world to live for." Yet the underlying concern is that her second daughter did not have enough faith in life or in the value of life itself.

ATHEISM IN THE FRONT PEW

On the whole, most of the people I talked with clearly recalled their religious socialization and the ways in which they moved easily into various levels of involvement with religion over the course of their lives. Some admitted to lapsed attendance for periods during their lives, while others described interpretations of theology, social teachings, and observances that were not a good fit with the official positions and practices of their various faiths. Thus, whether they were living independently in the community or in a long-term care facility, the older adults in the sample were keeping their faith in late life by adapting and redefining at least for themselves the problematic aspects of their faiths. People were not leaving or scuttling religion or their congregations, and they had, with eight exceptions, accepted doctrine without deep examination or reflection. Only a small number of people had come to their own terms with areas that concerned them.

Considering this prevailing tendency of adapting or working to reduce the gap between their individual understandings of religion and the institutional or official worlds of respective religions, it is of special interest to turn to four people in the sample who in most ways had redefined their understanding so thoroughly or who could not accept core elements of their faith, that the word atheist was used by them to describe their religious beliefs and how they viewed themselves. Again, the atheists were, in three instances, very active to moderately active members of their respective congregations.

Though his recognition of unbelief came as something of a surprise to Larry, a man with extensive and ongoing religious socialization, he stated matter-of-factly that he did not believe the Bible or even in Jesus. "I guess in some respects I may be an atheist. It's an interesting story [the Bible], but it hasn't made a believer out of me." Earlier he had said that what he actually believed in was the values of "a Christian way of life," but a Christian way of life that did not require a belief in God as a tenet of faith. His phrasing is consonant with the abstract idealism of Buddhism, which is centered on right attitude and right conduct rather than a deity.

Another man, Peter, described his experience with religion as "being raised on fear and guilt." Asked if other beliefs had replaced the Roman Catholic ones that had been inculcated, he said no. With various health problems that had recently intensified, he does not often attend mass these days. However, he remains a member of a parish. His epigraph on living and old age, "Any day above ground is a good day," was not offered in a humorous or sardonic tone. It was more a stark statement that life was found in basic survival. He did not believe in God and described himself as putting little effort into following religious practices that were once important to him.

Libby had the most extensive and complicated remarks concerning this. "Do I believe in God? I don't know. I'm open thinking about it. Maybe, maybe not. Do I believe in a personal God? Absolutely not. Absolutely not. Everything tells me there cannot be a personal God. What personal God would let a Holocaust happen? I mean, there may be a force. I suspect that the Oriental religions have the right idea. A whole universe that's one. Everything is an integral part of everything else. The microbes are part of us, and we're part of, 'we don't know what.' You know, I can see it that way. But a personal God, no. But people have a right to their religion. They have a right to believe in whatever they believe in. And what do I know?" She tells me that one of her children put it this way, " 'What kind of a God would need people to keep praising him?' If that's God, then who needs that? And I think that's true. So, as you repeat and repeat and repeat, the same stuff, particularly, in the Jewish service—I mean, you're saying the same thing over and over and over again. I keep on thinking, 'He's absolutely right.' What kind of a God needs this? On the other hand, . . . what do you do in shul? You turn around and you look at all the people. See who has a hat on. Who cares? . . . No, I wouldn't call myself religious. But I am respectful of all religions, and of all people's beliefs. That's why we have a Christmas tree. Because these little children [grandchildren] have their beliefs that they're being taught, and I'm respectful of it."

Alex shares these views about religion, "It doesn't mean anything to me. I don't believe in God. I don't believe it." I know he is on the call list for the minyan. When a tenth person is needed for worship, the synagogue calls him, and he reliably attends the service as the tenth man. Alex adds, "If they need the tenth person at the First Congregational—if they would call me, I would go. I would go because I feel needed, so I would go. But from a religious point of view—no, no, no. I don't know when I lost complete need for religion, but I lost it somewhere along the lines. I suppose we try to talk to our parents, you know?" He does not believe in God and with respect to prayer even during formal services he says, "No, I don't. No, I wouldn't say I pray, but I read the books. Every word has a meaning to me. It isn't that I read and it doesn't have any sense to me . . . [the words are comprehended] but to me, you know, I read and I say, 'What am I saying? To whom am I praying? What am I praying to? Who am I praying?' I don't go for Kaddish. . . . If they want me to come over, I'll be there. But that's about it." He tries to solve this dilemma by returning to the question of when this change occurred. "I don't know exactly when did it happen. There's no need for religion at all—no need, no need. It's funny because my sister went through the same thing I went through, but even worse. She believes in God. She does." I probe further about his support for the synagogue in the face of his own clear atheism, "But some things we support maybe because we are needed or because it's necessary . . . Necessary for other people. It's not necessary for me, but it's necessary—I see it. I can see it. Because some things are necessary for me, which are not necessary for some other people, you know?"

LATE LIFE TWEENERS: "SO, IN BETWEEN, I BELIEVE IN GOD"

There were four people who were similar to the atheists yet distinct from them in that they had questions about religious explanations and of particular theological dogma propounded in their congregations and by their faiths. It's not so much the case that these four were agnostic with an abstract seesawing about the existence of God; it is more that religious ideas were open to challenge. For example, two people attended and supported their respective congregations, but found that this act itself said or meant little in terms of people living ethically nor did it fit with scientific reasoning. Their view of religion was advanced from a more detached, intellectual stance. Thus, Phillip says that he tries to live a good life . . . "and if I see people not living a good life it annoys me." As to the importance of religion, "It's probably more important than I would acknowledge at first, because I think that's it's part of my upbringing, part of the way of life, and without religion think what we would be. So I mean, the impact of religion is very important. I am happy to acknowledge that."

Stephen says that religion was important to him when he was growing up. "But in recent years, I've become interested in the space program. Now I'm talking about two trillion planets and the universe is growing and it's shaking my faith. How could you, when you look at the entire sphere of things, the earth is so tiny and so, and then I've read the history of this planet where it was a hot planet at one time and how the oceans were formed and how life began and how plants began, and now we're talking about a man who created it in six days and rested on the seventh. So I'm not doing well at all in that department. I know there's some energy out there somewhere, but where and how and what, I don't know." He sums up "sometimes I've been tempted to believe that what we see is what it is." Stephen is also concerned about doing what is good. As a young man, he created his own daily prayer. He was on the road frequently, developing what would turn into a construction business that would become a leader in its field, and he wanted to start the morning "when I was working as a young man, my prayer every day was, . . . 'May I this day do what's right, say what's right, and think what's right.' That was my start of every workday. . . . They were words that I believed in. I didn't get that from anyone. That was what—I came from the old-type home where integrity was important, honesty was important and dependability was important. It was a home that was founded on those things, and you know those things, and you know they exist in spite of what's happening." In his home Stephen still keeps a copy of the "first New Testament that was given to me in Sunday school." Alongside it is his first dictionary. The imagery of these texts as neighbors after more than three quarters of a century, offers a compelling picture of the complex overlap between faith and intellect.

Wanda is included in this group of people who fluctuate between accepting tenets and reinterpreting them. She is clear on the core belief in God, "I believe there's a God, yes. I believe there's a God but I think what we have is a lot of our hell is here on earth, [chuckles], you know. Because when you go, when you die you're supposed to go where it's wonderful and no more sickness and all this stuff. How do you know? In fact, how do you know anything, you know? But I never thought of that until my brother died . . . I never thought of death. But when he died, it was such a shock." Wanda's observations are echoed in Joan's musings. "I don't understand too much, to tell you the truth, you know. But I believe in God. [laughs] Oh, yes. I believe in God. And that's why it makes me the way I am. Because everybody believes in God. So, I figure all the people that believe in God, they're all the same. It's a funny thing. Nobody came back from over there [heaven], you know, and tell us how it is and what's gotten them in. The only thing I don't understand is that God—why he allowed to have so many Jewish people murdered. Kids. Little kids. Suffering. They used to come around and grab the small kids out of your hands. And they used to cut their throat and stuff like that. Why does God allow things like that, if there is a God? So, in between, I believe in God, but I want to know where he is, and why he would do something like that."

OTHER MUSINGS ON THE MEANING OF RELIGION

Jean understood religion as "an inner thing" and something evident in daily life where it "shows up" in people "doing their everyday work." Jean used Mother Teresa as an example of a person who was religious. The relevant aspect is not the person or personality of this widely known and recognized religious leader, but the way her faith went to work each day with the poor. The unglamorous service on behalf of people is not so much the behavior to emulate for people in ordinary social settings, but the more general idea of moving belief into behavior in the very work individuals complete every day is the core of being religious. Well within reach of ordinary people, and an aspect of what came to mind in defining a religious person was the phrase "not harming anyone." This echo of Hippocrates is all the more instructive in that it comes from a person who worked throughout her life in the business of banking and finance.

Julia had this to say about defining a religious person: "I think they're all part of a religious person. I think if you don't care about your fellow man—you don't give a damn about what's going on—if your neighbor's

having a tough time—some people don't care, you know. They just
don't care! Even with my grandchildren—I mean, I care. But I've talked
to other grandmothers that say, 'Hey, that's their problem!' And don't
do a damn thing! But I know others that do just as much as I do, believe
me—and more."

Many people were reluctant to define or think of themselves as
religious people. When asked, many equivocated or even rejected the
term as valid for themselves. Mostly they demurred. Beth's response to
the question, "Would you call yourself a religious person?" is illustrative.
She replies, "I guess so. In that I believe in religion, I attend church,
and I do the best I can. I always ask the Lord to make me a good
person. Make me be a good person through the week." Similarly, Alice
hesitates about using the word religious for herself. "Oh, I think so. I
think so." She adds a supporting reference by emphasizing that "I taught
my children that way." The distinction she draws between being religious
and having faith is an interesting one. For her, faith means to "Be kind
to people, help people, and bring your family up right. My son—he's
married to a Jewish woman. He didn't have any children. He didn't
have any wife. He met this woman on a trip from work and he married
her. She's got her own children, and they get along good. Actually, we
celebrate Chanukah. . . . And they get along fine." The meaning and
value of faith is not automatically attached to any particular religion.
Religions differ in their expression of faith, but it is faith that is the
common denominator across religions.

Marilyn, a 78-year-old widow, reinforces the elemental and ordinary
dimensions of religion. "Religion matters in your everyday life. It matters
how you act. It matters how you treat other people, I think. I think it
helps you be—a better person." Edward notes an interesting aspect of
the distinction between a religious person and others, "You don't have
to belong to a religion to be a religious person . . . some people probably
need that group to keep their religion alive. If it wasn't for the group
they probably wouldn't have any [religion]. . . . If a person is good, let's
say he doesn't have a religion, but he's good [Ed defines good as
'kind, thoughtful, doesn't ask for anything back'] there's no difference
between a religious person and a good one except he don't have the
religion." Ed says religion made him "more caring." There is an implicit
recognition that practicing religion and keeping his faith sensitized
him to others in his family and others in his community of Laurelford
and increased the likelihood that he too might lend a hand to others
without expecting anything back.

Julia takes a different tack in thinking about this, "I think a truly religious person doesn't have to go to church every Sunday. And doesn't have to get all dressed up." For her, empathy, and being nonjudgmental about people who have troubles and difficulties gets to the heart of characterizing both a religious and spiritual person. As she considers the distinction between them, she says that they are "intertwined. I think they intertwine, all these things we are talking about today, they all intertwine.

Grace has lived for almost a half dozen years in a large publicly funded and subsidized housing project in Samuelson. She says, "It's getting better, but it was a mess at first. They've really improved it and gotten these roughnecks—kind of gotten them out of here." This view was supported by two other people I interviewed from the complex. Grace had some financial difficulties that resulted in repossession of her car and that encouraged her to move into the project. She thinks of herself as religious "because I go to church and I feel a good spirit." Yet she admits that "well we can have religion any way. Its [goodness] got to be within yourself . . . like some folks who don't even go to church." More important, she says that "religion gives me hope. Yes, you've got to have hope and justice." She was one of the few people in the study who explicitly linked religion [defined here as hope] with justice. Since she is a black woman from a childhood that featured education and practice in both Baptist and Roman Catholic traditions, it was not surprising to hear the theme of justice articulated. The surprise is that justice was mentioned by less than a handful of others as a component either of religion or of faith.

For Beth, worship is a central feature of what religion is, "Well, I imagine there are a lot of good people who aren't going to church, but I think church reminds you—it makes you think more about other people, and their needs and just brings it home to you. Things we need to be reminded of. Always having a good time [while attending church], no. I just think it's a good thing . . . I think church is necessary. I suppose people can be good. But I think they miss a lot [without attending]." This idea arises again as she defines a religious person as someone who has "kindness and compassion for other people. . . . It's probably harder to be a good person if you don't have the feeling that God knows how you—what you do and how you behave. . . . And if you don't believe in a higher power, God, whoever, it must be hard to be good. I don't know if people are born good, but it must be easier to stray if you're not religious, I should think."

Some link their weekly and formal religiosity with gratitude. Eugene, 82 years old, says, "Yes. I wouldn't want to miss or be late going to church. I think you have to give something back to the Lord for the week that you spent, you know? It's only fair that you do some return for the goodness of that week." Eugene considers himself religious because "I believe in God. I go to church. I say my prayers. What more do you expect?" He also adds that going to church helps him because it leaves him with a good feeling.

Nora describes herself in terms of religion as "Average, average religion. Not a religious fanatic, you know what I'm saying?" When asked about what characterizes a "religious person" she says, dedication, "I would say she's almost saintly, and that religion seems to be on her mind at all times, whereas mine wouldn't be at all times." Religion gives her, "Well, in my case it would be the strength to go on. To keep going. And to hope for the best. . . . I think that's peace of mind. I would hate to think that—if I had no religion, I'd hate to think—it would be a very vacant life for me. But that's me. I'd have an awful void—an empty feeling."

Robert says that attendance is central to his sense of faith. He attends church weekly without fail, "I don't believe in this two or three Sundays a year. Every Sunday I'm there. As a matter of fact, our service starts at ten. I'm at church at nine-thirty." His attitude and behavior is shared by 87-year-old Pauline, who has only missed church twice in 27 years. "Well, I feel as though if I miss church, my week don't go good. I mean, things just—everything is just so wonderful when I go to church. I have that wonderful feeling and I can't really explain how."

When asked about what she derives from religion, Lucy says: "I feel that it's a steadying force. It's certainly reinforced me. And it's enriched me through the fact that most of what I do has been involved around synagogue or when the children were ending day school, in particular, and I was very active in that, too. So, it's just a major part of my life. And it will probably be that way all the time. The Jewish Federation goes along with that, so I mean, it's Jewish identity, not that I go around preaching and what-have-you. But I'm very comfortable with it, and that's it. I feel more comfortable." She later adds "I think the sense of identity is most important to religion and answering the question, . . . by the grace of God, why am I here? And how can I be a good person? And I think this teaches us that if you study it, you can find out how we can better ourselves and do better to others in the world. That's the way I look at it."

Maxine offers this response to distinguishing between religious and good: "Let's put it this way. A person can be good without faith, but he or she can be more joyous and more secure if he or she does have faith. And I mean sincere faith. Not just fly-by-night kind of thing." She does not want to label herself as religious or spiritual—"Better to say, if possible, that I'm living as I think the Lord would want me to live. I do not dread the Big Tomorrow (death)."

As to the issue of separating being religious from being good, "Is there anybody that doesn't really believe in God? Really believe in God? There's a few that don't, but I think people can be good, but I don't believe that you'll be saved unless you confess to the Lord, Jesus Christ, that he's the son of God, and ask him to forgive your sins and save you. I believe that has to be done because—your goodness isn't going to save you." In response to how he would feel if he didn't get to church on Sunday, Hank, 80, said, "You're missing something. It's hard to put your finger on it, but it's like skipping dessert on a meal, actually. You're missing something."

Libby disavowed use of the word. "No. I would not consider myself religious. But I would consider myself respectful. We go to the orthodox shul because my husband is more at home in the orthodox shul. I, until [the former synagogue amalgamated], I maintained my membership for old times' sake, and I still send what I think are generous contributions in memory of my father's whole family, to the temple." She does not think of herself as spiritual either. "That's like giving yourself a pat on the back. . . . I'm very interested in ethical behavior and I hope that I'm ethical. I don't know about spiritual." And she adds, "I feel it's essential to belong—I really do. It's very important to belong to something."

Most people in the study did not and could not distinguish religion from spirituality, but Jack is one of the few people in the study who did. He characterizes the difference this way: "Religion is, as I know it, as I was taught and grew up in. Spirituality, I can connect to the entire, to the whole universe. I think there's a connection there. Religion is [more institutional]. Spirituality, I have a feeling that in the general workings of the universe, it might be there. Yes, I'm looking for an energy from the universe." As Maxine phrased it, "Religion is a part of living. It's a little like breathing. It's a natural thing."

RECKONING WITH CHANGE

"I have one nephew—I doubt that he's ever seen the inside of a church."

Nora comments on the relative absence of younger people from weekly participation and larger involvement in her congregation, but also sees that there is some carryover from the oldest generation's religious beliefs and behaviors. During her childhood, "of course, at home—the whole atmosphere was always—religion was always brought into our lives." There was "no choice." Indeed, as she observes, in the town in Ireland where she was raised, "everyone was a hundred percent Catholic, and we were. There was only just a few . . . outside the Catholic church." This is why she acknowledges younger people who participate in religion today. "And I give great credit to the people—the younger generation that do come to church, and I say, 'Thank God that they're going to church and following the appearance of showing thankfulness.' As they grow older, of course, it's up to them. They could follow it up or not." She recognizes in her own children's and grandchildren's lives that this culture and these times are very different from the world that shaped her childhood. When asked if she could see that the tenets and practice of a faith had been passed on to them, she replied, "Yes, I do to a certain extent because they both went to Catholic schools. They both went to Loyola High School. But then, they went their separate ways afterwards. . . . And I didn't question it because I felt, 'If they feel more comfortable in what they believe in, why should I be trouncing them with mine?' Because that can turn a person completely off. So, I left them alone. And I know that they know that the good Lord is with them, and that they have their own beliefs, and I don't question them— it's none of my business. And they don't harm anybody." She reiterated portions of this theme when generalizing about younger people and religious participation by saying, "they don't want to harm anybody. If they don't want to go [regularly attend services], that's all right. They have their own beliefs."

Robert wryly observed that "you don't hear anymore, as I used to hear as a kid, 'All right, Robert, get dressed. But put on your Sunday church clothes.' You don't hear that today." Robert recognizes and discusses the fact that his daughter's faith does not have what he calls the "depth" of his own in terms of membership, attendance, belonging. In addition, in terms of his grandchildren, the depth of commitment is not yet clear or certain. So there is a mixed set of results that older people see when they examine continuity and change in their own families and more generally in terms of the passage of generations. Allport's phrase "the mature sentiment" of religion may be an accurate shorthand for this ability to understand that generational change, as disruptive as it appears to be, does not signal catastrophe for faith.

Older adults have not yet concluded "that we are merely squandering the capital accumulated by our parents and grandparents. New religious sentiments are maturing all the time, producing fresh moral zeal, and engendering consistency upon men's purposes" (1960, p. 67). They see cause for optimism about younger generations and also cause for concern.

Many older adults were quite vociferous about the lack of respect displayed in the clothing worn to worship by younger people and their middle-aged parents. With respect to these visible changes, Walter decries the lax standards of attire for formal worship, as did virtually everyone else in the study. However, he also comments on the lack of affection he perceived in many religious or church-sponsored activities, especially for young people. "But you see, those are the things that I think the kids today are missing in church. You know, they go and they read scriptures to them, and that sort of thing. I don't know how they do it. I would love to sit in on a couple of classes, because if they have as much trouble with these kids as they do in the regular school—because I have friends that are schoolteachers—they're [religious institutions] on the edge. Every once in a while, I'll read an article where they say religion is coming back." He is not as sanguine about this as are the authors of those articles.

Pauline understands the particular changes and appreciates that there are signs of some small transmission of beliefs and behaviors. "I have a couple of kids [they are 60 years old or older] that—I won't say they don't like church, but they don't go to church. But I don't—I tell them that church should be their first thing to do. One of my sons, he was in the Marines, he said, 'Well, Ma, when I was in the Marines, we had to go church on Sunday, regardless.' He said, 'Now, that I'm not in the Marines, I don't have to.' But he takes me to church!" She is satisfied with the fact that despite less than conscientious formal participation, he willingly drives her to religious activities, thereby insuring that she can fully participate in the faith that is central to her life.

In the same vein as Pauline, Andrew and Lydia noted religion slipping away in the lives of their adult children. "We go every Sunday. I wish we could say the same thing about our family, but we can't." He talks about one daughter who has changed denomination and attends services but "not regularly . . . but that is no affair of ours, and we're very happy that they go to [to the new church]. They find faith in [a different] religion, and it's perfectly fine with us. No problem with that." Lydia added that another child and spouse "also attend" and belong to the same denomination, but lacked the "quiet fervor" that had been a source of belief and practice for her and Andrew.

Sometimes, older adults reflected on the changes in religious involvement that they had witnessed during the course of their own children's aging. Lucy, for instance, noted that some of the folkways of faith had been instilled in her adult children, "Nowhere near the same degree, but in different directions. The interest is, of course, still there. My daughter is always attending anything of a Jewish nature, as well as many other things. Very, very, varied interests. Our son surprised me most of all—our older son [who had lost interest when he was young]. But this is what I want to bring up. The surprise is that he is the most attached to it today. It's really astounding. He taught for 13 years in his reform synagogue. . . . He's the Chairman now. He said he had his Bar Mitzvah this year. Why? Because his son is 13, and he just had his Bar Mitzvah. So, my son said that after 13 years of teaching, he's tired of that weekend always being on a Sunday, having to teach school. He taught fifth grade Hebrew School for the synagogue, and . . . he never got reimbursed for that. But they like other things [now]. Mountain climbing, whatever else—they like weekends off." Lucy is gratified that some important elements of faith have survived across generations, and realistic about the press of social forces that impel a different direction and tone to its practice for her children and grandchildren.

Such diminution in commitment is a feature that older adults find pervasive among younger people in general. Speaking about intergenerational falloff in attendance and involvement by younger people in her own congregation, Lucy suggests that the length of the service might be modified a bit to accommodate the inelastic and scarce resource that time has become for younger people. "Probably, I think, that in keeping our younger people with our branch of Judaism, I would say one thing would be if it could be shortened a little bit. The service is long, and I find that my children balk over that [the service begins at nine and generally lasts two hours but may last until noon]. If there isn't a minyan, then the rabbi usually will use the time to teach us something, and he teaches us a blessing or something. But if they could shorten it a little bit, maybe it would be tolerated better by the younger people who just don't have the patience. Not only the younger, but I find, too, that among the older ones, they can't sit that long. They're anxious to, let's get through and let's get on with the program and keep on going. That's about the only thing that I can see that I would like to see change a little if they could just make it a little bit more—you know, speed it up so that it goes faster. I will say that in Israel, the services are over much quicker. Maybe they go faster. I don't know."

Among Jewish elders in the study, all discussed adult children and grandchildren, nieces and nephews, as having fallen away from keeping traditional practices that were still important to most elders, even if many of those practices were honored more in the breach rather than in practice in their own observance. In addition to a decline in formal participation, the domestic aspects of religion, for example, keeping kosher, or following established forms for celebration of major religious days like Passover and Yom Kippur have changed dramatically. With two exceptions, the elders were ambivalent about these changes. Sarah put it this way. "I kept kosher . . . my children don't. Because their husbands don't care. My husband didn't care, either, but I insisted." Nearly everyone had some direct experience of interfaith (Jewish and Christian) marriage within the corners of extended family, if not in their immediate family. The prevailing view was that this was a change that particular couples and their families had to "work out." Noticeably absent were philosophical or critical commentaries about broader implications or the impact on the religion or faith itself. For Libby and Alex, the inclusion of Christmas trees with the ornaments and music was open and celebratory, a way to acknowledge the value of grandchildren who were part of them in a way that went deeper than the nominal category or name of a faith.

Another grandmother who perceived similar currents of drift in the religious commitment in her family discussed this by using the image of "service roads in California, the ones off the freeways. You can go off on those service roads. You go on to them, but you don't get too far on them. The Christian life is a lot like that. We wander, we go off on a service road. So, we go off there and we wander around for a while. But when we decided that we're tired of that, we come back. And I always say, 'God is always right there when we come back.' He says, 'I was just here waiting for you to come back' [laughs]. So, I think young people do that, or people do." Later in the interview she returned to this idea in talking about younger people. "I suppose, as I grow older, I realize more what salvation or what living for God means, more than I did when I was young. I have a sympathy for young people because they don't realize what God means or they don't realize the seriousness of it. And there are so many temptations and things to attract them, that they are not close to God. But God understands. He reads the heart. He looks at the inner man, not the outward appearance. We look at the outward appearance."

Sally depicted this drifting away a bit more bluntly and concretely when she said of an oldest nephew, "I don't know that he's ever seen the inside of a church." Another very religiously committed elder, described younger family members in his extended family this way. "The younger ones have changed with the times. They get divorced and think it's perfectly legal, and they don't go to the priest and ask him for dispensation or anything like that, you know. They just go and move in and live with the girl, which in the old days, if my mother had, if my brothers or sisters ever did that, I think she'd shoot them; I think she would. Oh, she couldn't stand that."

Another view of the intergenerational changes in religious belief and behavior is expressed by Phillip. He talks about two of his adult children as having some concerted interest in religion and the other two as having been alienated by the Catholic church's position on independence in third world countries. The two disinterested adult children had direct involvement in the third world, one through the Peace Corps and the other from frequent visits to the sibling in the Peace Corps. "And I think that's what turned both our younger daughters off on the church and they've never really come back. I mean, they are friendly to the church but they are not active in the church." He uses a grandson's Bar Mitzvah as an illustration of the value of religion as a social glue and as an important source of clear examples of what is expected from young people and all people in terms of general standards of behavior. What makes religion appealing to him, he underscored several times in our interview, is not the rituals or theology; it's the historical perspective it offers to the understanding of culture and people. "That's what intrigues me about religion. It's not the strength of the religious feeling or the spirituality. It's more my interest in the study of its impact on history." He sees an appreciation for the historical perspective continuing in the third generation of his family. Later as we discuss some hymnals that belong to a nephew and are long overdue him, Phillip reiterates this theme in saying that he has "a number of old Bibles around which are important," for the "family and its history" as much as for any words of wisdom they may contain.

LOOKING AT THEMSELVES

Eugene thinks that there is a connection between old age and religion. "I suppose it seems more of the hereafter than we did before. When we were growing up as young men and women, we didn't think of that. We thought we were never going to die and never and never going to get old. We do now." He's a bit ambivalent about the future of religion. "It always will [have a place]. But maybe not as common as it is now, or not at all. But it was [it existed] years back. I think it will always be there some type of religion."

For Nora, age is connected to religion in the sense that she is more accepting of changes in life. She describes a "go with the flow" approach: "I do feel, though, that maybe I'm more broad-minded about things, that are associated with religion—that I'm more broad-minded about feeling that maybe, 'Well, if that's the way it is, that's the way it should be.' Or if religion doesn't improve [a situation], I'd say, 'Well, whatever is best. I think we'll get on with it,' you know. But I don't question it. So, I don't feel that it has changed my attitude that much, if you know what I mean. But I will accept what is. I'd be more accepting now than I was. At one time, I [when] very young, I couldn't accept the way it was supposed to be. That might be the only time that I felt that way. I'm a little bit more open-minded now about it. Maybe a little bit more liberal, maybe." She goes on to say that the changes in the church are agreeable to her. The new openness and acceptance in Catholicism are welcome. "Well, of course, you know some of those rules and regulations were made by the church not by the good Lord. I think now that they have come around to accepting what the people are comfortable with, rather than what they [clergy and church] were comfortable with."

When asked to comment on the idea that older people might have a special role to play or reach a unique stage in their belief because they were old, most were certain that older people in general did not have a special role. One elder summed up the collective pattern of response in this way. "I'm going to answer you in a funny way. I don't think that most people would be interested in anything they [older people] had to say. 'Oh, he's just some old goat. What does he know?' You know, all of us have our own thoughts, our own ideas, our own goals. And do we really care about what someone else wants or thinks or do they want to find God?" A few thought that local congregations might call upon older adults more frequently to teach about particular aspects of faith, but in the group as a whole there was not a strong sense that elders had something special to offer to their congregations or to younger people specifically. In these discussions a few elders remarked on their wish to have a "sound" understanding of other religions, not just their own. These few wished to receive more education about other faiths and were prepared to play the role of student and learner with respect to understanding other religions rather than to acquire the role of teacher within their own congregations or religions.

With respect to the relationship between old age and religiosity, Andrew thinks "that as people age, they're inclined to be more religious. But that's general, not one hundred percent, because there are people who will age and go to the ends of their days without too much thought of religion. . . . I think that generally speaking, age does bring on a feeling of—a stronger feeling of religion." Here he is alluding not so much to formal worship as to private thoughts and meditation about the meaning and purpose of life. When asked about the relationship between old age and religion, Lydia says "there's more time to appreciate what we have had, I think," not necessarily greater or more profound thoughts about the sacred but more time to reflect on the blessings and realities of living life.

Eric does not see a special connection between old age and religion. "I have no regrets that I'm getting older. I know my days are numbered. But I can honestly say, I can truthfully say, that I'm not afraid. You know, another Psalm that is always so great to me was Psalm 139, where God acknowledges you as an individual." He finds more meaning in this psalm today than when he was younger.

Gail sees that living and growing older have brought her even closer to her faith. She thinks her beliefs "well, I think that they have become stronger. Yeah, there have been changes because as a young adult, I kind of believe that I can do a lot of things myself. And even though I would pray occasionally, I felt a lot of what was happening, I could do. And I believe that after the 1960s and early 1970s, God has become more of a real entity, both stronger and more firm belief than I had as a younger person. And because of that, I can see more. I feel more certain that there is definitely a hereafter, and that there is still meaning in my life here. I feel more secure than I did as a younger person and my faith and my beliefs are basically the same, but stronger. Stronger, yeah. And more confirmed. Because, number one, I have more proof that it works, you know. When I was a kid, I didn't have the proof. I wasn't sure in 19__, that I would get my vision back, and they told me it wouldn't happen. But I do believe that because of prayer and because of positive thinking, because I think that makes a lot of difference, too. Thinking—you and your mind have got to be of one accord. You've got to be thinking positive to act positive. And the positive thinking plays a lot in things happening the way you want them to happen. Even though you may not actually do anything physically or directly to make it happen, but if you're thinking positive about something, and you're praying and asking God to intervene and you believe it's going to happen, then I think it works. But if you're wish-washy, and you're not sure if it's going to work, and you're thinking maybe somehow—hear people say, 'The Lord will make a way somehow.' No. The Lord will make a way, period. You know, never mind that somehow. I listen to people sing songs, and I don't think they really think of what they're saying. It's just that they like the rhythm. [laughs] No, the Lord will make a way, period. I put it in his hands and I trust and I believe it, it will work. And I think that this is what has happened over a period of years, is that I'm able to know that it's going to work. It may not work out the way I want it because not everything that I want for me may be what he wants for me. But according to his will, it will work out for the betterment of more than just me because I'm only one little entity—one little part—and it works out for more than me. Whoever it's going to help the most—people to have something positive go on, I believe that's how faith works. I think that it uses people in a way to make his world right."

Gail also acknowledges that much of a relationship between aging and religious belief depends on the individual and on the intrinsic nature of caring that the person has. " . . . People who are uncaring don't just become caring because they get older. They sometimes become harder and more negative. Because, 'Now I'm losing it' [getting older]. . . . It depends on the person from day one. I don't think that aging makes a lot of difference in a caring person. I think that a caring person—I've seen five-year-olds who have very caring personalities and who are concerned about something, and they care about people from the beginning. I think that uncaring people are uncaring. I don't care how old they get . . . I know more hateful old people than I do young people. They are just plain mean because they've just been mean. I don't think that makes a difference. I think that caring comes from inside and God gives it, and it's either there or it's not. I think that sometimes, as a person gets older, and they're no longer able—if they have a caring spirit anyway, and sometimes they're no longer able to be out and about and doing a lot of things, and they've been caring, I think that they might tend to be a little bit more generous toward helping because they don't have a need."

Much of the reckoning with changes in religiosity over time focused on two areas: 1) how younger generations had received the transmission of faith; and, 2) how the older person compared himself or herself against his or her earlier connections to religion. I now turn to a consideration of two theoretical concepts from adult development which have implications for the nature of religious belief and behavior in late life. The concepts treat late life as a unique stage of human development and posit the idea of a fundamental change in social perspective that comes from a turning inward, interiority, or from adopting a perspective toward others that is universal, gero-transcendence. Only a few older adults in the study provided accounts that are illustrative of these two features, interiority and gero-transcendence, that are thought to be associated with late life. Although interiority and gero-transcendence were pockets within the prevailing pattern of stable ties and practice of faith, they are emblematic of the underlying range of variation in religiosity. The concepts themselves have stimulated thinking and research in social gerontology and alert us to the internal and external processes that place individuals in different positions relative to religious experience.

INTERIORITY AND RELIGIOUS EXPERIENCE

A series of studies of community-dwelling older adults conducted in the 1950s, known to social gerontologists as the Kansas City Study of Adult Life, was a pioneer effort to understand processes of normal or typical aging. Members of the Committee on Human Development from the University of Chicago, with Bernice Neugarten as a principal force, set out to record the social and developmental markers featured in the lives of middle-aged and older adults. Most gerontologists continue to focus on issues of continuity and change no matter what the substantive topic is, but the Kansas City projects were undertaken with those objectives deliberately in mind. One of the patterns noted from the interviews, which gathered information about personality as well as social roles and activity in those roles or engagement, was a pronounced movement among some older adults away from an external, social orientation toward others to a pattern of "increasing interiority" in late life. Neugarten understood interiority to be related to ego and cognitive functions of personality which harnessed smaller amounts of available energy and shifted the locus of self-organization processes and the engagement of the older person away from previous levels of participation in social life and activities. Neugarten assessed this movement as

related to a decrease in impulse control among older adults and concluded from the data that this kind of interiority, a turning inward, was
not "directly reflected . . . until the mid-60s." She also noted that data
from other studies completed during the same historical period suggested that such a change in personality could be found as early as the
40s (Neugarten, 1963, p. 332). The finding of "increasing interiority"
among older adults was first embraced, then subjected to critical review
from a range of studies that found substantial support for activity theory
and from a theoretical confusion about the difference between social
structural vectors and social psychological processes of disengagement.
Though general social gerontological discourse has moved some distance from the concept, I return to it for this analysis because a few
people in the study revealed the kind of shift in their religious attachment that is consonant with "increasing interiority." Thus, the concept
may have a useful, heuristic value for this discussion and for thinking
about faith in late life. Remarks about social activities, including religious participation, as well as their accounts and stories about changes
in the level of engagement with others, all point to substantive and real
shifts away from broader social ties to a more inward looking and more
internally focused sense of self and identity. Such expressions about
lower levels of social and religious engagement reflected a marked
difference from earlier stages and ages of their lives—in a direction
consistent with Neugarten's original formulation of interiority. These
changes in orientation occurred among those who had high levels
of engagement previously and among those who had lower levels of
engagement during earlier years. The shifts are consistent with looking
inward, yet they are in some measure qualitatively and analytically distinct from other reflective processes such as life review (Butler, 1963)
or reminiscence (Birren & Deutchman, 1991). Again, the evidence for
interiority is direct and noteworthy, but as it is captured here it was not
characteristic of a great number of older adults in this study.

GERO-TRANSCENDENCE AND RELIGIOUS EXPERIENCE

In the opposite vein, a key feature for an equally small number of older
adults is the experience of gero-transcendence. This concept, which
like interiority is deeply rooted in social gerontology and adult development, was coined by Joan Erikson. She proposed a fourth adult develop-

mental stage or a ninth final stage to her husband's model of developmental sequences across the life course of an individual (Achenbaum & Modell, 1999). Gero-transcendence is described as a stage of "final maturity" that emerged from "withdrawal not wisdom" (Achenbaum & Modell, 1999, p. 25). In this regard, Erikson and Neugarten link their differing orientations to self and others to the same precipitating factor, diminishing biological and physical resources and the lack of energy characteristic of growing old. In gerontological circles the current word to capture this is frailty. In contrast to the outcome of interiority, Erikson posits a very different consequence to biological deficits associated with senescence. She contends that gero-transcendence may be a culminating stage of development in late life, "a surpassing of all human knowledge and experience," a period of possibility for an awareness of oneness with others and life itself. This quality of cosmic awareness and an appreciation for the mutable boundaries of human life—going beyond or transcendence of conventional boundaries—has sparked recent research into the concept by sociologists Robert Atchley (1999) and Lars Tornstam (1999). Specifically each has probed the concept with an eye toward offering ideas about measuring or operationalizing it and searching for some evidence of its existence among older adults.

Interiority and gero-transcendence are not broadly found as themes or orientations in people's lives as those lives are described in the face-to-face interviews. However, interiority and gero-transcendence are what I call "pockets" in late life experience; that is, they are found among only a few older adults but carry important insights into shifts of religious perspective, in interiority, or alternatively, gero-transcendence, that are uniquely associated with old age. Moreover, these two very different shifts in perspective have effects on religious and spiritual behavior.

GERO-TRANSCENDENCE

Even among the most active elders and those with high levels of religious involvement, there were subtle indications of shifts in perspective. Gail's observations about the necessity of moving to another level of faith in late life are illustrative of what gero-transcendence looks like—as a movement beyond the self at the same time that the person acknowledges that late life itself has the unique feature of a terminus. "I think that that's the whole key because if you—you can do all the talking in the world. But if you never put it into action, then you're not helping to foster, you're not helping to take care of God's creations, the things that he put here for us. And you can talk forever. But if you never do anything, if you just sit there waiting to die. You have got to do something, and teach. And I think that that's the key. You know, it's to be able to—even if you only tell one person something positive—that will help them out as to find an interest. Not necessarily find a life, but to find an interest in life. Because if you say something that would spark my mind, then I will go look for myself and try to find an answer. And I think that's one of the keys. You don't have to be sitting in church all the time, and you don't have to always pray—but you should be doing something to spread the belief in God."

Rose, 68, also illustrates a facet of gero-transcendence in her comments about how religion helps her these days. In simultaneous translation Rose says "that yes, her family helps her. But it's God that's really helping her and her family because she's always praying to God and asking God to help—not only her and her family, but everybody in the world. Those who are good and those who are bad because she doesn't believe that anybody is completely evil, that there's always a reason behind it. And that there's always good in everyone." This heightened awareness of others was underlined in other remarks. For example, some spoke about a change in how they placed the needs of others—others unknown to them—in a different light now that they were older. Such general awareness was often coupled to concrete behaviors like sending a donation, or participating in a group activity to meet a specific religious or humanitarian need. Jean said "I do think of others a lot. I think when you're younger it's not that you don't think of others, but you put yourself a little closer to the top of the list." She also noted that she is more generous in financial contributions now that she is not working.

Other examples of the varied forms that gero-transcendence may take are evident in the accounts and experiences described by Anne and Jack. Their observations provide a sense of the concept's richness, not so much a literal or concrete example of what gero-transcendence means, but how it plays out in their lives. Anne was a religious searcher, ahead of her time. Her religious experiences map out the kind of personal searching detailed in *The Five Stages of the Soul* by Moody and Carroll (1997) and in the searching of younger Boomers, described by sociologist Clark Roof (1993, 1999). Her present religiosity is centered around a heightened awareness or transpersonal bond with others. It has taken her a lifetime of spiritual searching, filled with twists and turns, before she reached a point of understanding that seems consonant with Joan Erikson's concept of gero-transcendence. At the time of the interview, Anne was living in Chelsea Court's independent unit. She had recently encountered a number of serious health problems. Though most of them had been resolved through surgery and long-term recuperation, these health problems required continuing levels of assistance in a long-term care setting. She continued to receive some daily assistance with household tasks, but had improved in terms of health. During the course of our long interview, Anne spoke at length of the spiritual journey that had threaded through her life, from her days in high school through cross-country moves, a divorce, and the uncertainties of raising children on her own at a time when one held a pariah status for doing so. Anne had reached a level of oneness with others some years ago when she actively sought out different religions and different traditions in order to move to a faith that understood the dilemmas of divorce—one that did not cast the divorced person's spirituality into a void. Her extensive contact with other traditions as well as the education she obtained brought her almost full circle in terms of her religious identification today. But as she stated emphatically, it was not the "religion itself that was important, it was the realization that after all, we were one." It is this higher level of spiritual understanding that defines her life as meaningful even though she now resides in a long-term care setting with institutional ties to the faith that had excluded her and her children many years ago. She follows her present faith, but also uses the dedicated religious spaces of a former faith for daily meditation. She is also conscientious about attending formal services offered two or three times a week by her former faith. She reads widely about a range of religions and hopes to take classes at a nearby college now that her physical health and strength have been recovered.

At 85, Jack was among the oldest men in the sample. I literally bumped into him not long ago as he was entering and I was exiting a local health food restaurant and store. He is among the most fashionably dressed elders, dapper and stylish. Denim and sweatshirts have not ever found their way into his closet. He talked extensively about the narrow meaning that the traditional forms of faith and observance have for him now. He is increasingly drawn to a different level of understanding about the meaning of life and man's relationship to God. He commented on the findings from physics and astronomy—findings about the universe that shed new light on our purpose here as human beings. This was not the kind of talk that would endear him to the majority of his local congregation, nor is it the kind of talk he would think of expressing to them or others. He noted how his growing awareness of the limitations inherent in conventional understandings of faith and the very definition of God had sparked new ways of thinking about spirituality and consciousness. Like the majority of those I talked with, his was and is a deeply rooted engagement with faith, but the fundamental concerns he has had since his wife's death several years ago have taken him in a new and much different direction. He appreciates and is exploring new ideas about the universe and the divine with a wide range of reading and with some fellow travelers. This takes him worlds away from his weekly worship. His is an erudite and thoughtful search that was moving him even further along the transpersonal dimension of being at one with others. In one sense this is an extension of concerns he has had for most of his mid to late life. He has, for example, been a major and anonymous donor to several area school scholarships as well as a community philanthropist to other charitable efforts, all without a nameplate. The gero-transcendence here is one of increasing depth and doing even more with respect to supporting others at the same time that his thinking and reading have led him to perceptions of the permeable and gossamer boundaries between science and faith. During the formal interview he showed me the more "socially oriented" book he had just begun reading; it was *Bowling Alone.*

INTERIORITY

Ellen is 90 years old, single, well educated, with a long career in the private sector in a position that marked her as a pioneer. When I interviewed her at Chelsea Court, she was still making an adjustment to her relatively new surroundings. About three weeks before she had been moved here from her own home because she required a higher level of nursing care. She was experiencing problems with walking. She had previously lived alone in her own home and recognized that she would not return there. A relative had just made arrangements for a closing on her house. It was as she said "on the market three days and poof, sold." She was surprised, but she already had a better setting in mind, an assisted living facility in the same town, and she expressed what seemed to be genuine confidence in her relative's ability to take care of these things. He was called "a lifeline."

Many of the details about Ellen's faith and life suggested that for some time she had been drifting away from active engagement and was now looking inward for the sources of faith and the beliefs that would help her move through this acute health crisis. She had been raised in Christian Science and still found those teachings and principles to be mainstays of her current reading and thinking. She had been a member of only one congregation many years ago and it was not a Christian Science congregation. Since then she had not maintained a formal membership in any congregation. She told me that she found great insight and comfort in the books she now kept in her small bedside table, but the communal activity and formal membership had faded as she grew older and now were nonexistent. The intellectual aspects of Christian Science principles were, however, important to her and she maintained them through reading that literature as well as from her other secular reading. Her subscription list was extensive and she managed to keep the current, social world before her, at a distance to be sure, but there. Unsurprisingly, and reinforcing Neugarten's original linkage of health and interiority, Ellen's acute health problems were gently pushing her orientation further inward, but had not yet altered her hope or capacity to see a personal future.

Larry's discussion of life was frank. He was seriously ill. There is no clearer illustration of interiority found in the sample. When we talked, it was as though Larry was peeling away every social tie to life, ties that had once been rich with meaning. It is difficult to say whether these ties were falling away or to what extent Larry was actively stripping them away. As was the case for many of the men in the sample, Larry was a veteran of World War II who returned home to complete education that soon led to a white-collar occupation in the financial sector. He progressed upward and retired in the 1980s. In childhood and throughout his life, religion was always important to him and he was a full-fledged participant in a local congregation, doing everything he could throughout the years to assist the minister and members. There wasn't a position he hadn't held or task he hadn't done for the congregation. Yet when we talked, it was starkly clear that aside from disengaging from lawn work, housework, and the more onerous aspects of belonging to a congregation, Larry had moved to dead center. He was looking inward to such an extent, that golf, and just socializing with longtime male friends were among the ties that had fallen away. He was, I think, as solitary and reflective as any elder I've ever talked with who was facing the initial phases of life's passing away while he was still looking on. Interiority was a kind of sanctuary for him, a place safely away from people where he could reflect on the ending that was close and for which the folkways of faith had lost the capacity to explain.

In the foregoing examples of elders whose lives reflected aspects of gero-transcendence and interiority, there is much to weigh in terms of links to religion. This chapter discloses the subtle ways that older adults change their perspectives on religion and faith. There is evidence of reckoning with changes that brush up against late life complacency from younger generations, culture, and religions themselves. Though members of the study have stayed the course, there are a few who move in separate streams toward the horizon. As Victoria, 90, said, "I think sometimes on what it [religion] all means. There have been so many changes in what we [Roman Catholics] do. But I go and give praise not knowing if what's changed ever really mattered, but when we were young it sure did." Most people in the study moved as Victoria did with the folkways and the changes prescribed by the religions. Only a few moved ahead or apart from the folkways of their religions.

CHAPTER SIX

Folkways of Faith in Long-Term Care Settings: Self, Soul, and Space

"Religion is the finding thing. I could never live without it. Today I went at 10 because the sister she'll say, 'you're coming to mass with me'... not that I didn't want to go."

LONG-TERM CARE SETTINGS AS SOCIAL WORLDS

Older adults residing in long-term care settings share in many of the folkways surrounding faith and religion that are described in earlier chapters. Their words and experiences are not separate from the words and experiences of community-dwelling older adults. Both groups of older adults practice folkways of faith in similar ways and both groups find private prayer to be the touchstone of daily practice. Nevertheless, the residential settings of long-term care facilities, the structures and social contexts constructed for care, anchor the individual socially into a qualitatively different social world and set of experiences with respect to living life including a life that has some attachment to religion. The particular features of each institution have much to do with how an older adult puts religion into practice. Even in the less restrictive settings of retirement communities, this point is driven home. In a qualitative analysis, McFadden (1999) traces the correspondence and thoughts of John Casteel as he encounters the difficulties with activating his faith within this setting. His writing, both journals and letters, does more to keep his faith and spirituality alive than do many of the religious events sponsored for the older residents. His letters reveal the arid and forced nature of many religious activities. The letters record the frustration that comes from having a meaningful faith blocked and evince the resolve that leads him to find some expression of this faith through the words and interaction of correspondence.

There has been an increase in awareness about the responsibilities institutions face in recognizing religious issues, and new attention has been drawn to the matters of faith among institutional residents with Alzheimer's (Wentroble, 1999) and other diseases that impair a range of cognitive and physical functions. Yet the literature that records the view from inside these social worlds has consistently highlighted a number of themes that press us to examine the obdurate reality that remains a part and parcel of long-term care (Diamond, 1990; Gubrium, 1993; Lidz, Fischer, & Arnold, 1992; Savishinsky, 1991; Shield, 1988). Though there has been progress in opening up what Goffman (1961) called "total institutions," there is considerable room for improvement with respect to enhancing individual autonomy and to making dependency a bearable predicament (Lustbader, 1991) if it is not one that can be alleviated through human effort. This chapter recounts some of the special features of folkways of faith identified by older adults in long-term care and it presents information about the settings and the ways in which staff and the institutions offered pathways for participation in faith. As is the case with many issues, long-term care facilities draw our attention to their work and efforts precisely because they are among those entities by which we evaluate our own record as a culture and nation. As Heschel (1981, p. 32) originally phrased it, "The test of a people is how it behaves toward the old. It is easy to love children. Even tyrants and dictators make a point of being fond of children. But the affection and care for the old, the incurable, the helpless, are the true gold mines of a people." It is in this spirit that some special features affecting folkways of faith in long-term care are presented as they emerged from the interviews with residents.

SOME CHARACTERISTICS OF PEOPLE IN THE LONG-TERM CARE SUBSET

Consistent with national data on nursing home residents, people interviewed in the long-term care facilities were older than their counterparts in the community-dwelling sample. The mean age for the entire group was 83; the men had a mean age of 77 and the women had a mean age of 86. Based on visual assessment of gait, posture, and ease of movement within the area of the interview, the oldest among the institutional group were more frail than were their counterparts in the community sample. Based on verbal fluency, memory, language, interaction, and the ability to move through the interview process, there were no gross differences between the long-term care group and the community sample with respect to cognitive ability or in recall and response with respect to topics covered in the interview. Inasmuch as the study did not examine or measure cognitive impairment, and considering that one person was in the first stage of Alzheimer's disease, and another had experienced some psychological problems, the interviews proceeded well, without any unexpected or out of the ordinary turns, only the missed cues and beats that are part of the usual flow of conversations and interviews. A hint of difference between the long-term care and community-dwelling older adults appears in the average length of time for the interview. Long-term care interviews were typically shorter by about 10 minutes. There were interviews in this group that were long, two hours and longer (the shortest interview in the study was with a community-dwelling respondent), but this time differential does suggest that both person and interviewer gauged and adjusted their conversation in response to elements that were unique to the interaction and situation.

People in the long-term care subset were not significantly different from the community elders in terms of most social characteristics or in the range of the background characteristics from early childhood and family experiences. Two uniform features in the long-term group that made it different from the community-dwelling group were that of ethnic background: people were from a mix of western, northern, southern, and eastern Europe cultures, there were no ethnic minorities interviewed in the long-term care group; and that of health status, which was associated either with vulnerability to an assorted range of acute problems or with a diffuse frailty in addition to the presence of at least one significant, chronic health problem, e.g., multiple sclerosis, cardiovascular disease, or various forms of cancer. This latter feature is likely associated with the fact that the long-term care group was slightly older than the community-dwelling group. However, one of the most striking features noted previously about the community-dwelling group was also characteristic of the long-term care group—they were lifelong or nearly lifelong residents of the state, and also, in most cases, of the larger town or city where their long-term care residence was located. The magnitude of this stability of residence in terms of forging social connectedness and a buffer for major disruptions in life is not to be understated. One person from Daphne Lane, took me to a window to point out a home, less than a block away, that had been a lifelong residence. Such close proximity to the place where one's life had un-folded, was in this case, a source of comfort and pride to the person.

THE LONG-TERM CARE FACILITIES

The six long-term care facilities or nursing homes that make up the institutional subset of this community study of religion in late life were sites for 15 of the 46 interviews. Interviews with older adults and limited observational work occurred in five of these facilities, while a sixth nursing home was the site for participant observation. The facilities were chosen because they varied in size (as indicated by the total number of beds) and with respect to the kind of ownership of the facility (i.e., profit/nonprofit status; religious or secular affiliation). Increasingly ownership, even of religiously-based long-term care facilities, is subject to issues of corporate control or to management practices that are guided by overarching business and financial considerations and con-cerns. However, with respect to the institutional or cultural ethos, it was thought that long-term care facilities with longstanding ties to religious groups or organizations might also be places where a deeper level of concern for the individual and for matters of faith would be displayed. Last, although it may be described as stating the obvious, the facilities were also selected on the basis of their willingness to participate in a social science research study. It was clear from the outset that each nursing home had a slightly different historical role in the larger com-munity and that there were local cultures within each institution that had differing ties to the larger cities and towns where the institutions were located. Each institution, in a distinctive way, was open to the idea of participating in the study and was aware of the boundaries that separated the researcher from the daily work they did to provide health care and residence. Each facility was helpful about providing practical and logistical assistance and in permitting the researcher to fill the role of a visitor with a specific set of research objectives. The institutions, in every case, adopted a laissez-faire approach or neutral stance with regard to the study once the researcher fulfilled the particular review procedures with appropriate staff members at the facility. Two facilities (the largest ones) had well-educated and experienced staff members whose roles in the facility called upon them to understand research

processes and procedures and from time to time to work with researchers. One long-term care facility had a full-fledged and efficient internal,
institutional review board (IRB), more knowledgeable and savvy about
ethical issues than many a research university. There was tremendous
variation in the steps necessary for the researcher to follow in order to
secure permission to talk with older residents about their lives as well
as their religious beliefs and behaviors. Such variability was onerous in
the sense that each site had unique expectations and wide-ranging ideas
about the nature of the social scientific research process (though all
seemed to be better acquainted with medical models for research).
Staff members had various levels of familiarity with issues regarding
privacy and interviewing. This is a roundabout way of saying that acquir-
ing permission to conduct interviews involved a great deal of interaction
and preparatory work. To a certain extent this is unremarkable and
reasonable for qualitative research particularly as it speaks to the role
of an outside researcher unknown to institutional personnel whose
study was based on face-to-face conversations with members of a group
(the elderly) defined by federal statutes as a protected class. I was
not using methods based on disguised or nonparticipant observation.
However, I often wondered as I crossed institutional thresholds just
how cognizant residents were of the fact that by living in these settings,
their ability to say yes or no to a wide range of social activity was limited
and constrained by social forces unseen to them. Often during my
observations, and only in the kindest ways, I noticed that the adult
status of the residents was not fully endorsed by staff members so much
as it was paternalistically protected. It was as though the parietal hours
of colleges and universities, the ones that were scuttled in the late 1960s
and early 1970s, had found a new roost in present-day long-term care
facilities. This may be just the kind of social barricade that the first
wave of aging Boomers will have the energy and experience to tackle
in their old age.

It is fair to say that while the institutional setting was not widely
admired or acclaimed, and residents were not fully aware of some
aspects of their confined environment, by the same token, the people
I talked with were not unduly concerned with restrictions on free association or their range of choices. Some expressed chagrin and resignation
about their limited mobility and the small stage for the play of daily
life. Like the character Norma Desmond from the film *Sunset Boulevard*,
residents of long-term care facilities did not see themselves as shrinking
with the passage of time; instead the size of the screen and the stage

for their lives had become much smaller, particularly in the nursing home. Some of them noticed this and had objections to it. Most understood that their move into institutions was a consequence of changes that had come into their lives as a result of their own difficulties with health and the frailties of advanced old age. They perceived themselves as having faced and addressed those issues by moving from the community to the institution. However, most also understood that some part of the constraints and adjustments they made were also part of "the system." There were programs of interest, but there were also limits to what the long-term care facility could provide. A few did not find services and programs that adequately met their needs. The complex set of events that brought them into long-term care and the relationship and weight of these events were acknowledged if not always accepted by people living in long-term care facilities.

As stated earlier, but a statement that bears repetition, the names I created and gave to the facilities are pseudonyms. The names are not representative of the settings nor are they meant to evoke any symbolism. They are simply handy place names for the residential buildings and property that comprised a long-term care facility. Having said this, I must note for readers that long-term care facilities often have names that are bland, chosen, one supposes, for their ability to elicit nothing other than a vague image of a typical street address. Alternatively, a smaller number of institutions are directly and clearly linked to a religious tradition and are accordingly named. Nevertheless, there is a vast common ground in terms of names. For example, other than saints' names or the names of religions, there is little use of the names of exemplary public, civic, or otherwise widely known or esteemed people. The names I applied to the facilities follow in the tradition just described and are as follows: Chelsea Court, Daphne Lane, Ivy Corner, Maple Way, White Pines, and Chestnut Grove. Any similarity of names to actual facilities is coincidental. As far as I can ascertain, there are no institutions with these precise names in the state of Connecticut.

Overall, the six facilities had physical and social settings that were not grim or bleak though each facility was unmistakably institutional. By institutional I refer to the intended function of the space and its subsequent layout and design. Facilities were meant to meet health care needs and needs for daily sustenance of older people provided by a trained staff in a quasi-self-contained, separate system. Thus, anything remotely homely is an adaptation or improvisation to the general design scheme and structure of the facilities. The term, nursing home, though used in this book interchangeably with long-term care facility, and with the word, institution, remains a euphemism speaking more to the intent than to the reality of life for residents. Likewise, after several visits to individual institutions my impressions are favorable with respect to sanitation and to the general, visible, upkeep of the facilities and their grounds. This observation is all the more notable because the facilities themselves (with one exception) were older, some dating to the early twentieth century, and, in the language of the building trades, the oldest among them had been retrofitted and renovated either entirely or substantially in order to provide long-term care or to implement new techniques and technologies associated with changes in the nature and magnitude of skilled nursing care. Moreover, the trend in institutional care over the past decade has been for the elderly to be admitted at increasingly advanced chronological ages and in poorer health, which means that there is more labor and expense related to health care as well as to maintenance and housekeeping than was routine even as recently as a decade ago. I also observed a fair amount of equipment in each room I visited. The spacious places were the corridors.

Though no one I interviewed was happy to be living in a facility, all concurred that the basic level of amenities was adequate. "This isn't the Ritz," as one man put it. That sentiment was echoed in less evocative language used by other residents. This statement was often linked to the thought that the person had not, of course, lived in such grand quarters as the Ritz before becoming ill and frail and "ending up in this place." But home had been home, and no matter how one tried to view the nursing home as a lateral move, there was no honest way to equate a room or half of a room with the space in the homes people had left behind. There were less than a handful of people who had plants or pets in their immediate living area (this seemed to be the result of limited size and space as well as other factors). People also had an assortment of suggestions for what and how some specific aspects of living could be improved, but most were resigned to the space and the place. As one person put it, "Where else can I go, now that I am like this?" Another 96-year-old pragmatist declared, "I don't like it here. But you've got to make the best of it." When I asked if there was one thing she would change about the nursing home, she laughed and said, "I'd get out of here!" Then after a slight pause she added, "But I have no place to go."

For a handful of the older women, this rhetorical question, "Where else can I go?" was explicitly connected to an awareness that this particular nursing home was their last or final home. Barbara is direct and realistic about her residence at Daphne Lane: "When you come in here, you're going out feet first. Don't think that I think anything else. I don't. And that's the way it's got to be." Barbara has arranged for her funeral and burial and is not so much preoccupied with death as clear-eyed about its eventuality. She has survived a number of strokes and has experienced a substantial loss of physical mobility, and to some degree, her recuperative capacity. She is also an illustration of the kinds of movement, changes in residence, that shape the lives of others in long-term care. She, for example, had made at least three residential moves during the last decade. In her case each move was to a nursing home with higher levels of medical care. Another pattern related to changes in residency is that the men had moved even more frequently and had been residents within the institutional setting for a slightly longer time than the women even though the men were as a group younger than the women. This hint at gender differences may be related to variation in health status as well as to the existence of a broader network of social support for women that works harder or is somehow able to keep them in their own homes for a longer period of time.

The facilities themselves varied in terms of several social structural dimensions including total size (buildings and grounds), the total number of beds, and the physical layout of the residential units and within the residential units. These variables are detailed in Appendix A. Only 2 of the 15 people interviewed in the long-term care institutions officially had a private room; 13 shared their rooms with a roommate, and at the time of the interview, a few did not have a roommate. In many cases, residents and their roommates shared their quarters with some fairly sophisticated yet space-greedy pieces of technology. When the machines themselves were absent (signifying better health of the occupants), accessories like mobile trays and other portable equipment still occupied a substantial amount of space in the room. This spatial dominance of necessary equipment has the effect of reinforcing the more mechanical if not inhospitable aspects of life within the rooms. Unlike prison cells with unobtrusive video and other surveillance equipment for monitoring inmate lives, the nursing home rooms were filled with equipment to support life although life itself was being crowded out by that very apparatus. Moreover, from a broader perspective, each facility was constrained by the reality of physical structure and layout. It is not the case that design and form follow function carefully and with keen attention to detail in these versions of dormitories sans campus.

Buildings themselves were both planned and unplanned; that is to say that even when they were purposely built for long-term care, the lag between planning for the population of the building and filling the building with treatments, practices, and people gave rise to the problematic reality that each facility from its inception could not project or live up to the needs or uses it was pressed to deliver at the turn of the twenty-first century.

In a real sense the facilities, although never authentic homes, have made strides toward achieving some ambience of a homelike atmosphere, if not a cozy one, even with an array of technological support (respirators, other mechanical equipment) that is largely absent from the private residences of community-dwelling older adults interviewed in the study. Crossing the threshold into these six long-term care residences was akin to having the experience of déjà vu, in that each institution is a distinct social setting with a special history and particular emphasis or purpose, but each is similar to the others in that the facility and institutional culture come to dominate the individuals who work and live there.

SPATIAL AND SOCIAL DIMENSIONS OF THE SACRED

One important theme that emerged from the interviews in long-term care settings and from observations in the facilities is the nature and meaning of space, and the creation and definition of sacred space in a facility. Having such space, private and shared space, as well as having the ability to use such space, may be crucial to the continuous practice of faith and to its expression in the daily lives of residents. A central principle for all religions is that there are places and times that are sacred, imbued with the divine, and therefore special in terms of the behaviors and ideas evoked by use of that space. Related to space, and perhaps of equal importance within long-term care or institutional settings are two other factors: 1) the role other social actors, residents, and staff play in enhancing or limiting acts or expressions of religious belief and behavior; and 2) the opportunity to participate in group and individual experiences that support religious expression as well as a broader sense of well-being.

Erving Goffman's (1961) concept of the total institution speaks directly and usefully to the general institutional context in which these 15 elders lived. Some important features of total institutions are identified below.

- The physical separation of the institution from other parts of the community
- Restricted mobility and access to the institution from the world outside its doors
- Limited access and mobility for residents within the institution
- A trained staff as the arbiters and monitors of social activity within the institution; knowledge of the rules, authority, and power to interpret and implement them is found among staff members

Decades after he wrote extensively about total institutions, it is mildly surprising to note how widely applicable Goffman's concept remains to an analysis of contemporary long-term care facilities. The distinctive physical and social worlds of long-term care facilities are set off by the social and physical boundaries between the institution and the community. Just a short visit to a nursing home is enough to remind a researcher of the degree to which mobility is restricted: check-in points for identification; double-check for caution; and, in some places escorts are provided. All of this is polite and civil, not rude or boorish. Indeed, given the move toward safety and security that has driven many changes in how outsiders are treated and processed in a wide variety of other institutional settings such as courtrooms and public schools, settings that are more "open" as institutions, one could suggest that the model of total institutions has come to be taken for granted even in public and civic settings for interaction.

The nature and quality of sacred space (space for religious activity and interaction) cannot be set apart from general issues of controlling movement and limiting access to space within the walls of the long-term care institution. Institutional space is not open or available in the sense of being unrestricted. Hence the ability to use it, or if it is not built-in or what is often called, a dedicated space in the facility, to find or create sacred space, is likely to be influenced by the ethos and spirit of the facility as it is expressed in staff behavior and in staff response to the elderly residents of the institution as much as it is influenced by the number of square feet administrators can find for such activity. This also suggests that individual concerns or social patterns of the residents may not influence the ways in which the sacred finds space on the floors within the institution.

FEATURES OF THE LONG-TERM CARE FACILITIES

In the next few pages, some brief descriptions of the facilities present a glimpse of their material and social circumstances. This is not intended to give a comprehensive description, it merely places or points out how the facilities fit within a larger context and informs the discussion about space and religious observance and practice.

CHELSEA COURT, RELIGIOUS AFFILIATION

This large facility has a deeply rooted history and visible presence in the suburban community where it is located. Like Ivy Corner it offers a range of care and is understood to have a religious affiliation. This is visible within the structure, and residents or would-be residents are well aware of this feature, though one need not be of any particular faith to be a resident.

CHESTNUT GROVE, SECULAR

This small facility was designed to provide long-term care and had a rather unique design that appeared to facilitate somewhat different interaction among residents and between staff and residents. It was found in the same small city as Daphne Lane.

DAPHNE LANE, RELIGIOUS AFFILIATION

A midsized facility with an official religious affiliation, but one that was not as immediately visible as Ivy Corner or Chelsea Court. A major part of the physical structure was dedicated to long-term care, but there were other buildings with service and programs for other groups of people. Located in a small city, the facility itself had a long history of serving as a site for social services.

IVY CORNER, RELIGIOUS AFFILIATION

This is a large institution with deep roots in the community and state. The institution has formal ties with a mainstream religion and though one does not have to be a practicing member of the religion to become a resident, the formal religious ties are part of the social world and culture of the place. The religious tie is visible and widely understood and recognized. Thus it is not a surprise to find that other aspects of the organization of the facility include institutional compliance with religious-based guidelines and visible symbols of the faith. Ivy Corner is also acknowledged as a local and regional leader in research related to long-term care.

MAPLE WAY, SECULAR

A small facility in one of the state's major cities with noncorporate, secular ownership and no formal ties to education or research. This facility was the most urban in terms of its location within one of the state's largest cities. Indeed, five of the six long-term care facilities were in urban or medium-sized suburbs; only one was found in a small community that had once been agricultural but is now suburban.

WHITE PINES, SECULAR

A midsized, nonreligious facility with independent corporate ownership and a formal link with a nearby health facility that was once a community hospital. Indeed, at a time when the community hospital was in sound fiscal condition, White Pines was built across from the hospital's main parking lot. Some crossover or migration between populations was anticipated and incorporated into the design and placement of the White Pines building.

SOME INSTITUTIONAL DIMENSIONS OF SACRED SPACE

BUILT INTO THE STRUCTURE: IVY CORNER, CHELSEA COURT

Space was defined and planned for religious activity at the outset because of official and formal ties to a religion (not necessarily a particular religious organization but to a religious and theological belief system). Part of building and design was to dedicate distinct and special places for religious activity of residents and, later on, as an adaptation to needs of others, chiefly staff and visitors. Planning and reserving facility space assures at minimum that use of religious space is not compromised or given over to other activities. The space also is special in the sense that it is consecrated. This does not, however, assure high or consistent rates of use. Like the experience of larger freestanding community religious congregations, designing and reserving dedicated sacred space does not mean that people will use the space or do so in a consistent fashion. Building sacred space into a facility does not assure that "they will come." No "Field of Dreams" is to be found here.

ADAPTATION OF EXISTING SPACE

Chestnut Grove, Daphne Lane, Maple Way, and White Pines were facilities that adapted and improvised when sacred space was to be found for religious or devotional activities. This improvisation occurred in a number of ways.

INDIVIDUAL AND INTERPERSONAL DIMENSIONS FOR ADAPTATION OF SPACE

This pattern occurred when space was found jointly through interpersonal interaction. Here, secular space was periodically adapted for sacred activities. Residents and staff arranged space for religious use and adjusted in creative ways to the absence of separate, dedicated space for this purpose. People made over secular spaces like multipurpose rooms as they regularly transformed them into religious spaces for specific periods of time. Multipurpose spaces have an eerie generic emptiness that is transformed only when human social activity occurs within their walls. If one photographed the life of such a room in a time-lapse series, the contrast between the nondescript rooms and the livelier moments of certain activities including prayers, devotions, and a range of other activities would be compelling. Such a time-lapse series would understate the labor-intensive efforts needed to bring people together for any purpose including sacred or religious ones.

SPACE FOUND SPONTANEOUSLY AT CHESTNUT GROVE

At Chestnut Grove, in part due to its unique design, I observed a spillover from formal boundaries into common areas created by individuals. Hallways and corridors are generally places to see and be seen. Here during a memorable set of observations I noticed that in the hour before lunch people often moved into areas near the corridors and fashioned an "as if" front porch from which they watched comings and goings. I also noted that several people carried with them visible symbols of religion such as prayer books or rosaries, and a few, in the pauses of mainly staff comings and goings, read portions from their books, some vocalizing or almost reading out loud. This was in the larger colorless and flat interior walkway a rather lively, spontaneous activity. The whys and the wherefores of how this came about might shape another project; suffice it to say that the residents who peppered the hallways and perched their wheelchairs so they could see and be seen, offer some small proof that light and warmth can come from people in spontaneous, human ways. For just a moment in time they changed the meaning of the corridors albeit temporarily by using the tiniest spot of institutional space in original ways, ways far removed from design or function.

ADAPTATION OF EXISTING SPACE THROUGH RELIANCE ON STAFF

Because common areas or open rooms in larger facilities have multiple uses, adaptation of space quite often means horrific logistical and scheduling arrangements that require staff initiation and support of sacred activities. Moreover, in one's own room, whether private or shared, assistance is needed to move and tend objects and religious calendars, posters, statues, prints, documents, icons, and photographs from visits to holy sites, and to assure that medical equipment and ease of access for staff (food, cleaning, PT, OT, etc.) have priority. Despite these real challenges, I observed that three of the elders had arranged their living areas in such a way that in each room there was a kind of sacred ambience radiating from the arranged material items that they valued. These places were tiny fractions of their allotted space in the room for a bit of the sacred—a corner or small wall area, the top ledge of a television set graced by statues and religious cards, a set of passages taped to a bedstand—just enough to make a connection with faith and with identity. Cohen and Moore (1999, p. 100) describe a similar, but more purposefully designed space within residents' rooms as "the religious corner." To see this, whether by design or innovation, encourages the consideration of how such sacred spaces might be placed within long-term care facilities.

FINDING SOLITARY SACRED OR SECULAR SPACE IN THE FACILITY

Fortunately, individual expression of faith may require only modest, even smaller areas of space, than those discussed above. Logically one may ask, How much room does a person need to have a place to sit; a bit of quiet for reflection and prayer? The objective answer is that a few square feet will suffice, yet it is precisely these private, retreat spaces, sacred or secular, of a few feet which are the most difficult to find or to arrange for within institutions. Though multipurpose rooms are at least available though perhaps difficult to access, individual sections of shared rooms, that is to say living space, are relatively small. There is only room for a few visible items of display, and the local culture of institutions seems to mitigate against what might be termed either clutter or liveliness of individual preferences for décor.

Not surprisingly, visible representations of saints and of Jesus Christ were found displayed in several of the residents' living areas. One reproduction of the Holy Family was displayed. Other religious motifs included calendars (not exclusively in English), religious cards, various styles of crosses, some small but recognizable statues, some prints, and two iconographic depictions (I did not observe any crucifixes). Among Jewish residents whose faith traditions do not support representational religious depictions, there were far fewer items of faith displayed or featured in personal living areas.

One striking electric Chanukah menorah (candles violate fire codes) was featured in Ruth's room (the interview took place shortly after Chanukah). Ruth was pleased to have it on loan. "Yes. This menorah also belongs to the Sisterhood. [A member] brought the menorah back and—I don't know why the red color is there—last year we had white bulbs. They were so beautiful, and they all were lit." Ruth was one of the only people to leave a long-term facility regularly in order to attend formal worship services. She depended on friends from her synagogue (which had been joined with another synagogue) to provide rides for her. As she tells me, "These people that I see there are mostly the generation in their 70s." She manages to attend services regularly but not as often as she once did. She has experienced increasing difficulty with hearing and that has interfered with the pleasure she once had in listening to the rabbi's "wisdom." She is convinced that if she could but sit in the men's section of this orthodox shul that she would be closer to the rabbi and hear him. She'd like to be able to do that, but says it wouldn't be possible.

Other reminders of Jewish identity that are not necessarily indicative of religious beliefs or folkways of faith were found. Small but visible pieces of Judaica were clearly displayed, a Magen David of glass or crystal, a chai placed on the wall. It is important to note that among the Christians and Jews in long-term care facilities the visible reminders of belief and identity were found alongside similar items associated with family and the individual's life.

The necessity and organizational imperative of monitoring inhabitants leads infrequently to actual examples of solitary space, and perhaps rarer still, aesthetically pleasing private space, particularly among long-term care facilities that feature assisted living and skilled nursing care. This is also the kind and quality of space that is well-nigh impossible for residents to create spontaneously or as part of joint action with staff members. If small quiet niches aren't built into space from the start, it is difficult for anyone to create them after residents are in place.

ONE PERSON'S EXPERIENCE AND USE OF SPACE LEADS TO A STRONGER FAITH

As was noted in chapters 3 and 4, the folkways of faith found among older adults were not influenced strongly by residential setting. In order to speak to the broader issue of space in the lives of residents in long-term care, James's experiences and adjustments offer a good illustration of the continuity of these folkways and the real changes that people make in this setting in order to keep those folkways.

James was raised in an actively religious and nationally prominent extended family and has lived in Chelsea Court for a few years. His grandfather and father were both mentioned as significant in his development of faith, a faith whose denomination changed from Methodist to Roman Catholic when he was nine. James and his wife were active members of a Roman Catholic parish. His wife's untimely death 10 years ago confirmed his faith rather than altered the course of his belief. A parish priest was able to arrive in time to administer last rites to his wife. This fortunate occurrence gave him something to take away from an unexpected and sad loss. He says "these kinds of events test people's faith, but it made my faith stronger."

An earlier test of faith for both of them had been their inability to have children. The death of an infant they had been hoping to adopt and for whom they had completed the paperwork and preparations for adoption was a blow that they absorbed by understanding that it was part of a plan with a meaning that could not be understood by them. Their faith and their extended family are credited with moving them along in life even without having had children of their own. James also sees his faith from childhood as profoundly connected to formal worship and ritual. He adds that having mass "available" three times a week is very important to him. He regularly attends because it is an opportunity to pray and to get "closer to God." Despite the fact that others (two brothers-in-law) "quit" the church after the Vatican II reforms, James never considered that. The one religious item he keeps in his room is a cross, now hanging on his refrigerator, but awaiting some help from a nephew to hang it in a "better place." He also keeps his mother's Methodist Bible.

He is aware from his own experience of the decline in religious vocations. He continues to read books about his faith and talks about changes in the church. He watches some contemporary religious television programs and attends the Sunday mass in his electric wheelchair, which he likes very much (I can attest to this personally as I witnessed him on noninterview days zipping along the corridors). It allows him to get into the balcony, which he likes because it's not as crowded as the main floor. He also relates a story about attending a black fundamentalist service which interested him deeply: "And I thought to myself, 'Boy, I wish I could be as close to God as these people are,' . . . it's a different approach, a different expression of the relationship." His prayer practice is full and he credits Chelsea Court with fostering this. Indeed, he may be becoming altogether too other-worldly, as he wound up the interview by telling me that he has to settle his cable account or he would lose his connection with television.

He's also aware of how scarce men are in the nursing home. To a certain extent he finds this flattering, but he also says that he misses the company and friendship that men would add to his life. He ends with a story about the Methodist church in New York City where he first attended Sunday school in the time before he became Catholic. "[They] bought the church and turned it into a mosque . . . a couple of my friends went back to see it and they called me up and told me all about it . . . to become a mosque, but that's what's happening." His surprise and appreciation for the changes in religion were expressed in tones of honest amazement. Not many people spoke in terms of their faith becoming stronger; James was actually the only person in the entire sample to discuss religion, spirituality, and belief in this way.

His behavior matched his statements and for him there was a clear strengthening of what had been a line of identity; it was now an all-encompassing one.

ADAPTATION TO PLACE AND SITUATION: CONSISTENT FORMAL ENGAGEMENT

Another long-term care resident, Marie, exemplifies a similar connection to formal engagement with religion over the course of her long life. With eight grades of schooling provided by a religious order and a family steeped in religious participation and membership, Marie describes her faith then and now as "natural." When asked about the most important thing she has taken away from religion, Marie, without a pause replies, "Well, I've never taken anything away. I took it in." Important as her faith has always been, Marie admits that it was even more important during a time of great personal trouble in the aftermath of a horrific fire that occurred several decades ago (O'Nan, 2000). In the kind of vivid detail that belies the half century passage of time, Marie recounts the events of that afternoon, which left her hospitalized for a year. In retelling what happened, Marie describes the horror not of her own serious burns and injuries, but of witnessing the death of others. A woman Marie had been talking with at the time the spiral of flame began its descent "down the sides of the tent," froze in her seat and was "charred to death." The suffering defies reason and the point is not that Marie invokes any religious explanation; in fact, she does not. Rather the point is that the tragedy does not make her more or less religious, as she said about religion itself earlier, she takes it in. She prays and attends religious services in the long-term care facility. In commenting on the importance of religion to understanding life and other people she says, "I think religion goes the full way, all the way through."

Douglas is another nursing home resident. He was born and raised in Maine in a Roman Catholic household with both parents from French-Canadian ethnic backgrounds. After the family's move to Connecticut, they became members of a French-Canadian parish. As an adult he was a lifelong member of another Roman Catholic parish. His sense of religion is one of practical participation, "I felt that it was my duty to go to church, to go to mass." He does not attend a formal worship service in the facility where he resides. He does, however, participate regularly in a devotional group organized and conducted by a minister. He finds that group helpful and says that "I try to learn because I don't know the Bible." He also says "That's what I'm getting out of this group. Me reminiscing on what's happening [in the passages discussed] and reflecting on what I heard when I was small which is forgotten." He attends major holiday worship services (Christmas, Easter) but finds the group reading and discussion meaningful, so much so that later in the interview he adds spontaneously, "I enjoy the religious studies I wish though, we don't have enough people anymore . . . because nobody's available. A couple stayed and they'd fall asleep or they're not well." The group itself is small and "some of those people are just not ready. We had, when I first came here [10 years ago], we had more alert patients but now . . . what we're getting is a lot of real sick older people." Thus the happy existence of a regular and meaningful program for residents is influenced by larger structural issues. As he says, the biggest issue is that "there's not enough challenge here."

Patrick is a lifelong resident of the larger community where the nursing home he now lives in is located. He cannot attend mass now and misses it, but has prayer books and other books that he reads and finds helpful. When asked about the role of the Eucharistic minister, "Well, he just comes in and gives you Communion and there's nothing. You just say the prayers that you'd normally say." Religion, prayer, and reading are important. Like Douglas, Patrick participates in a devotional group and looks forward to the reading and discussion, "you know a little more about your religion than when you started." He is also aware of the fact that other residents are often unable to participate in these or other activities because they respond in different languages to English prayers, or behave inappropriately for the setting.

Barbara keeps up active and regular contact with the clergy and some fellow parishioners and remains a member of the congregation though she attends services offered in her long-term care facility. Like Douglas and Patrick, Barbara participates in a devotional group, a Bible study group. She talks favorably about the ordination of women and says that "I always knew I could call God when I needed him." Margaret is another long-term care resident who participates in a devotional group. She finds it helpful and looks forward to it. She credits the group leader for caring about the members and working through passages from the Bible and from other sources. She appreciates the group because "their system, their singing, their thoughts and everything about it is very inspirational to me." The group, under the highly motivated direction of one staff member, had adapted a multipurpose room in order to hold their daily morning discussions. The space and the surroundings were less important than the social and religious activity, listening to religious affirmations, offering prayers, listening and responding to the staff member's discussion of a sacred passage, singing, and listening to recorded music. The fact that a community Sunday service was held regularly and that residents could arrange to attend the service provided Margaret with an additional opportunity and a more familiar ritual for weekly religious observance. Nevertheless, the hour-long devotional did daily duty in reminding people of their special purpose even in this institution and with all the difficulties they faced. She concludes by saying "Oh, I enjoy it so much. And I have never missed [the leader's] sessions."

CONCLUSION

Speaking of losing track of time in the facility, and more generally, of her sense of life during the last year, Margaret says, "Then, when I came here, you lose track. You don't know what day—you have to ask people sometimes, 'Is today Saturday?' [laughs] 'Or is it Sunday?' It's an entirely different way of living, dear. Entirely different." The residential and institutional space that surrounds older adults in long-term care was recognized by more than a few as a place from which they would depart "horizontally." Despite this sobering reality and the press of countless other reminders that there was little room for autonomy and even self-expression in their last homes, older adults were as active in prayer as their community-dwelling counterparts, but less involved in following some of the folkways of faith. For example, several people attended formal worship within the facility, one or two attended services outside the facility, and several had given up attendance entirely. Some of this drop-off in the interactional aspect of religion was linked to health, but some is related to the lack of sacred space within facilities. When smaller devotional groups were offered in the facilities, a number of people attended and found their participation to be enjoyable and helpful. The interaction and the substance of the readings was much anticipated and meaningful. Yet in order to find the space for what I call, devotional groups, the staff had to work creatively through other program schedules and activities in order to use space that was designed to be multipurpose, but like one-size-fits-all, ends up by not fitting well with most activities.

It is also possible to stimulate more of the sociability that is tied up with living in groups, particularly the penchant for displaying meaningful items that speak to the religious and spiritual dimensions of identity. However, I suspect the conundrum underlying the absence of small private and small but larger intimate spaces (those suitable for 8–10 people) is as much a matter of bricks and mortar, money and politics (specifically how we decide to spend socially generated monies), hence, largely intractable. The good news is that residents and staff are improvising and have managed to create some activities that stretch the soul along with other parts of the self. Meanwhile, people in long-term care continue to offer thanks for all that is wonderful in life and to express that gratitude without regard to place. I can almost hear their refrain to these lines from "Welcome Morning" by Anne Sexton.

> so while I think of it,
> let me paint a thank-you on my palm
> for this God, this laughter of the morning.

CHAPTER SEVEN

Conclusion: Beyond a Reflexive Faith?

"Religion is not for the weak-minded. It's the strong-minded person that can stay with God and stay close to God. You've got to be strong-minded because there's so many things to draw you away now."
—Clara's rebuttal to a widely quoted, public statement made about religion by a Minnesota governor

"I believe in God. I go to church. I say my prayers. What more do you expect?"
—Eugene

"It makes me feel that I belong to something, and I belong some-where. I mean, none of us are here for no reason at all."
—Walter

REFLEXIVE AND REFLECTIVE DIMENSIONS OF FAITH

For most older adults in this study, the religious beliefs and the folkways of faith which are an important part of their lives are reflexive. Folkways, as is true of all effective customary ways of doing things, including religious practices, direct people into specific behaviors and patterns of behavior without the need for them to give that behavior a second thought. There is no need for contemplation or imagination when cultures and social institutions provide folkways and norms. Eugene summarizes the main dimensions of reflexive religious behavior in the second quotation above: a belief in God, conscientious formal worship, and the most significant part, prayer. He adds the rhetorical question,

"What more do you expect?" This is a fair question and a probing one. If, as various scholars and writers have contended, there are special tasks in late life, such as significant well-being, gero-transcendence, ego integrity, life review, acquisition of wisdom, and as I suggest here, the development of a reflective faith, the answer to Eugene's query is, yes, a little bit more is expected and needed. The little bit more is not in the direction of a fanaticism or exclusive concentration on religion, something that most people in the study understood to be a misdirection in terms of faith. But a little bit more is expected in terms of stretching the soul, and in so doing, stretching the self and identity.

Regardless of the particular theological requirements or definitions of soul, stretching the soul, or moving beyond the usual and accepted patterns of faith—that is, doing religion with more than conformity to sturdy folkways—necessitates reflection. Thinking, deliberately and deeply, considering the ideas, tenets, and actions that are part of religion and of one's faith, how best to manifest the insights gained from such reflection, all are pieces of a reflective faith. A huge leap or break with folkways is unnecessary but a stretch is expected in order to stay sharp and to avoid complacency about elements like justice and transcendence. These components of faith have roots in most religions, yet it was curious to note how few members of the study expressed concerns about the reflective dimensions.

But is this asking too much of faith and of older adults? Traditional folkways of faith may serve well despite the lack of reflection. Steinsaltz, for example, points out that "perhaps even the vast majority of people, can also reach a very high level of spiritual being. It is possible, even, within the confines of the available, overt tradition. A person has simply to worship God with love and fear" (1988, p. 272). However, Steinsaltz also calls habit a "dilemma" for religion. The dilemma may be posed in stark terms for people such as religious leaders and thinkers, social gerontologists, and theorists of adult development who analyze and study religious behavior and its place in the course of life. The dilemma may be a matter of perception in that it is associated with prescriptive views that posit challenges and tasks for ages and stages of life. Mastery of these challenges and of other intellectual and religious ones are viewed as welcome instances of growth. This may be more of an artifact of theoretical and analytic frameworks and not an authentic part of the lives of older adults, or a stage associated with late life.

Reflexive faith is adequate to the challenges many people in the sample faced as they moved through life and through old age. Reflexive

faith and its folkways were meaningful. Nonetheless, there were periph-
eral and sometimes central issues that were left unresolved and subject
to musings, doubts, and questions. What was identified as missing from
religion, even among those with a reflexive faith, was an understanding
of some of the more complex mysteries of life. Sunday sermons were
not sound sources of explanation for questions that people had about
the reasons for suffering, the meaning of witnessing the pain of any
number of situations that people encounter. People who posed such
questions, ones that might be expected of a mature faith, did not find
ways within their faith to move to a reflective stance or to seek answers.
This lacuna may be significant to explore.

Another interesting feature of reflexive religion is that in this sample,
at least, there was a lack of certain forms of the instrumental use of
religion. A few people observed that the instrumental value of religion,
the idea that church or synagogue was part of worldly "business," such
as a way to make connections or sales, was off-putting. Though a few
people described some attempts to use prayer as a way to assure a
particular instrumental outcome, they dropped this approach rather
quickly because they understood more reflexively than reflectively that
prayer did not work in this way. Most often prayers were of petition
rather than of transcendence, although there were also prayers of gratitude and praise.

In terms of cohort succession, this pre-World War II generation did
not seek accolades because they had been steadfast in faith. Indeed,
they wondered aloud and were puzzled about what it was that they
could usefully transmit to younger cohorts, including some of their
own elderly children and younger but adult grandchildren, about the
value and meaning of religion and faith. After all, nearly everyone
recognized how much different the world was today. In fact, this rooted-
ness or stability in terms of geographic or residential status was another
unique feature of the group. There was a high level of social mobility
in terms of education, occupational status, and income, even among
the oldest of the women, but with a handful of exceptions, people were
rooted in the state. Moreover, they also said that the sense of belonging,
established in their own lives decades ago, was a most important part
of what faith meant. This theme had more depth to it than the equally
widespread belief in God. In fact with respect to the latter, there were
several who expressed doubt. Yet that doubt did not keep doubters
from the social obligations of belonging, that is, participating in congregations or faith or in supporting them.

This picture changes focus when the long-term care setting is considered. The fifteen people interviewed in this subset of the study all agreed that religious involvement was important to them. For two people there had been a change from previous levels of participation. In these two instances, the structure and organization of the nursing home played some role in the change, but a lack of mobility and restricted access to religious space or to clergy were not primary factors in their disinterest. Having said that, it became very clear from the interviews and the observations within the facilities that space and access to space posed some issues for religious practice. The space and access issues could be partially surmounted by the wild-card of caring staff members, paid and unpaid, who were enthusiastic about offering programs to residents. I observed one such program on two occasions and found in comments from participants that the program was appreciated and a high point of the day. Leaving less to serendipity were the three facilities that provided dedicated space for religious activities and had some cadre of paid and unpaid staff to support religious and devotional activities. Here, the issue was twofold: residents had to be engaged in ways that were meaningful to them, and the physical mobility of residents affected the logistics of moving people to the dedicated space for religious activities. The positive feature of the six facilities was that each was aware of both the merit of providing access to religious activities and the responsibility to meet some of the religious and spiritual needs of residents. The difficulties encountered were in some sense cemented into the institutional arrangement that Goffman so many years ago aptly called total. The challenge faced by staff in institutions is not insurmountable, but it is daunting. Four of the six facilities relied on a physical layout that was not designed to absorb social tasks that the facility sought to accommodate. In addition, the absolute paucity of private space in every facility does not augur well for encouraging the reflective or reflexive private prayer that older adults valued and practiced or the creation of that comfortable spot for a talk with God.

The overarching and ongoing linkages of social ties to others—in both groups—the long-term care residents and community-dwelling older adults, was a connection based upon kinship and ties to proximate generation adults; sons, daughters, nieces, and nephews; with significant ties often superseding those to age peers; spouses, siblings, and friends. Adult grandchildren were significant for at least two of the elders interviewed, but this tie was often more talked about than it was real in the daily lives of the majority of older adults. A close affective tie with the third generation was spoken about, yet overall this tie and perceived relationships with grandchildren constituted a familial reference group more than a primary group. The central figures for frequent interpersonal interaction, including religious and spiritual activities, were age peers followed by second generation even though some among this group were also elderly themselves. Why is this important to note? In terms of religious and spiritual life the interior work and the exterior work of keeping the faith were framed by minimal contact with younger people. In virtually all of the settings, direct contact with religious persons was with middle-aged or older adults. This centering of faith as a real-time activity in late life means for the most part (even in congregations) that interaction is within rather than between age groups or generations. Though congregations may take as an article of faith that religious practice and ritual moves across generations, there is in the interviews a clear depiction of interaction with respect to religion that is age-concentrated and homogamous. People do not speak of knowing or maintaining contact with younger congregants unless those congregants are very active participants in formal or recognized religious groups within the larger church. Thus, when members of a congregation visit elders in long-term care settings the visitors are themselves elderly or middle-aged members from the former religious community.

Gutmann's (1987) discussion of the impact deculturation has on the elderly and the buffer traditional cultures place between the old and the fractured folkways of urbanized societies offers both a psychodynamic and an anthropological perspective on the value of preserving such niches and creating what he calls "developmental milieus." The people interviewed in this study appeared to have staved off the effects of deculturation, in part because most had backgrounds built on stable residence in the state. They carry with them the features of having been socialized in patterns that mimic traditional societies. In a sociological sense this is significant and may speak to the larger issue of adequate adjustment to the transitions of aging and to the substantial losses people had experienced. With respect to the long-term care group this pattern is also clear. Continuous, lengthy residence permits the evolution of an attachment to place over time, such that one is connected biographically in a way that is qualitatively different from the more ephemeral connections that are found among the newly arrived, in this case, those people with less than a quarter of a century in the state. The length of life spent within a community is a robust measure of the ability to carry on with activities and interactions that are part of late life and to participate in new social milieu (Eisenhandler, 1994). And even for those who immigrated across international boundaries in younger, perhaps as late as early adult years, the stability of community placement is, I think, a kind of social innoculant. These older adults were not wanderers nor were they alienated or dislocated by larger social forces. They had experienced some of the effects of social change, but they spoke about themselves and others with the assurance of knowing their bailiwick well. Older adults here were centered and able, despite other kinds of losses and difficulties, including residential moves of less than voluntary origin to long-term care facilities, to sustain customary social behaviors and beliefs because they had residential stability and biographical security. This means, for example, that for most of their lives bumping up against age differentiation was a feature of daily life within the context of a circumscribed and familiar community. With respect to religious and spiritual beliefs and behaviors this means that although a few departed directly and significantly from the traditions of their parents, their own religious socialization was generally of the same shape as that of their parents. It was also the one they passed on to their children, but they observe that the world has changed, and that the impact of religion had been altered for younger cohorts.

As endings always turn on their beginnings, I return to the oral histories collected by the Federal Writers' Project to conclude with a statement from an interview in the 1930s with an older adult, Andrew Jonas. "Some of the Burns Chapel brothers come for me and Ma on Sundays, so we can get to church. I sure love goin' to meetin'. Looks like there's a heap of comfort in religion, and I shore believe in prayer. I aim to make out just the best I can, and put my trust in the Lord" (Federal Writers' Project, 1975, p. 355). The passing of the 20th century and of the generation born before World War II will soon be followed by the folkways of faith or of other beliefs that characterize the young-old among the Baby Boom generation. This generation may trust in the Lord, but the idea of Lord and the ways of trusting have changed. How the succession of faith will manifest itself is unclear. Yet the basic orientation or social imperative toward transcendence is likely to emerge in new forms if, as Simmel said, "the attempt is made to conceive of life as something which constantly reaches beyond limits toward its beyond and which finds its essence in this reaching beyond" (Simmel, 1971, p. 373). Keeping folkways of faith will extend the possibility for reaching beyond, and there may be new folkways emerging to foster transcendence and reflection as old and young generations continue their journey through time.

References

Achenbaum, W. A., & Modell, S. M. (1999). Joan and Erik Erikson and Sarah and Abraham: Parallel awakenings in the long shadow of wisdom and faith. In L. E. Thomas & S. A. Eisenhandler (Eds.), *Religion, belief, and spirituality in late life* (pp. 13–32). New York: Springer.

Allport, G. (1960). *The individual and his religion.* New York: Macmillan.

Atchley, R. C. (1999). *Continuity and adaptation in aging: Creating positive experiences.* Baltimore: Johns Hopkins.

Augustine, S. (1961). *Confessions.* (R. S. Pine-Coffin, Trans.). Middlesex, England: Penguin.

Birren, J. E., & Deutchman, D. E. (1991). *Guiding autobiography groups for older adults.* Baltimore: Johns Hopkins.

Blumer, H. J. (1969). Society as symbolic interaction. In J. G. Manis & B. N. Meltzer (Eds.), *Symbolic interaction: A reader in social psychology* (pp. 139–148). Boston: Allyn and Bacon.

Buhler, C., & Massarik, F. (1968). *The course of human life.* New York: Springer.

Butler, R. N. (1963). The life review: An interpretation of reminiscence in the aged. *Psychiatry, 26,* 65–76.

Cohen, U., & Moore, K. D. (1999). Integrating cultural heritage into assisted-living environments. In B. Schwarz & R. Brent (Eds.), *Aging, autonomy, and architecture: Advances in assisted living* (pp. 90–109). Baltimore: Johns Hopkins.

Coles, R. (1975). *The old ones of New Mexico.* Garden City, NY: Anchor Books.

Copland, A. (1985). *What to listen for in music.* New York: McGraw-Hill. (Revised edition of 1957 original work)

Deland, M. (1911). *Autobiography of an elderly woman.* Boston: Houghton Mifflin.

Diamond, T. (1990). Nursing homes as trouble. In E. K. Abel & M. K. Nelson (Eds.), *Circles of care: Work and identity in women's lives* (pp. 173–187). Albany: State University of New York Press.

Durkheim, E. (1965). *The elementary forms of religious life* (J. W. Swain, Trans.). New York: The Free Press. (Original work published in 1915)

Eisenhandler, S. A. (1994). A social milieu for spirituality in the lives of older adults. In L. E. Thomas & S. A. Eisenhandler (Eds.), *Aging and the religious dimension* (pp. 133–145). Westport, CT: Auburn.

Elder, G. H., Jr. (1974). *Children of the great depression.* Chicago: University of Chicago Press.

Ellis, A. (1985). *The case against religion: A psychotherapist's view and the case against religiosity.* Austin, TX: American Atheist Press.

Erikson, E. H. (1963). *Childhood and society* (second edition). New York: W. W. Norton.

Federal Writers' Project. (1975). *These are our lives.* New York: W. W. Norton. (Original work published in 1939)

Fowler, J. W. (1981). *Stages of faith: The psychology of human development and the quest for meaning.* San Francisco: Harper and Row.

Frankl, V. E. (1963). *Man's search for meaning.* New York: Simon and Schuster.

Freud, S. (1964). *The future of an illusion* (J. Strachey, Ed. & W. D. Robson-Scott, Trans.). Garden City, NY: Doubleday. (Original work first translated and published in 1927)

Gavron, D. (2000). *The kibbutz: Awakening from utopia.* Lanham, MD: Rowman & Littlefield.

Gergen, K. J. (1991). *The saturated self: Dilemmas of identity in contemporary life.* New York: Basic Books.

Goffman, E. (1961). *Asylums.* Garden City, New York: Anchor.

Gould, R. M. (1978). *Transformations.* New York: Simon and Schuster.

Gubrium, J. F. (1993). *Speaking of life: Horizons of meaning for nursing home residents.* New York: Aldine de Gruyter.

Gutmann, D. (1987). *Reclaimed powers: Toward a new psychology of men and women in later life.* New York: Basic Books.

Hewitt, J. P., & Stokes, R. (1975). Disclaimers. *American Sociological Review, 40,* 1–11.

Heschel, A. J. (1981). The older person and the family in the perspective of Jewish tradition. In C. LeFevre & P. LeFevre (Eds.), *Aging and the human spirit: A reader in religion and gerontology* (pp. 35–44). Chicago: Exploration Press.

Idler, E. I. (1994). *Cohesiveness and coherence: Religion and the health of the elderly.* New York: Garland.

James, W. (1929). *The varieties of religious experience: A study in human nature.* New York: The Modern Library. (Original lectures delivered 1901–1902)

James, W. (1963). *Psychology.* Greenwich, CT: Fawcett. (Based on 1890 two-volume Principles of Psychology)

Kierkegaard, S. (1962). *Works of love* (H. Hong & E. Hong, Trans.). New York: Harper and Row. (Original work published in 1847)

Koenig, H. (Ed.). (1998). *Handbook of religion and mental health.* New York: Academic Press.

LeClercq, J. (1982). *The love of learning and the desire for God* (C. Misrahi, Trans.). New York: Fordham University Press.

Levinson, D. J. (1978). *The seasons of a man's life.* New York: Knopf.

Lidz, C. W., Fischer, L., & Arnold, R. M. (1992). *The erosion of autonomy in long-term care.* New York: Oxford University Press.

Liebow, E. (1993). *Tell them who I am: The lives of homeless women.* New York: The Free Press.

Lifton, R. J. (1993). *The protean self: Human resilience in an age of fragmentation.* New York: Basic Books.

Luke, H. M. (1987). *Old age: Journey into simplicity.* New York: Bell Tower.

Luke, H. M. (1995). *The way of woman.* New York: Image.

Lustbader, W. (1991). *Counting on kindness: The dilemmas of dependency.* New York: The Free Press.

Mannheim, K. (1952). The problem of generations. In P. Kecskemeti (Ed.), *Essays in the sociology of knowledge* (pp. 276–322). New York: Oxford University Press.

Marinier, P. (1954). Reflections on prayer: Its causes and its psychophysical effects. In P. A. Sorokin (Ed.), *Forms and techniques of altruistic and spiritual growth* (pp. 145–164). Boston: Beacon Press.

Mathews, M. M. (Ed.). (1951). *A dictionary of Americanisms: On historical principles.* Chicago: University of Chicago Press.

McFadden, S. H. (1999). Surprised by joy and burdened by age: The journal and letters of John Casteel. In L. E. Thomas & S. A. Eisenhandler (Eds.), *Religion, belief, and spirituality in late life* (pp. 137–149). New York: Springer.

Mead, G. H. (1964). *George Herbert Mead: On social psychology* (A. Strauss, Ed.). Chicago: University of Chicago Press.

Mead, M. (1975). *Blackberry winter: My earlier years.* New York: Pocket Books.

Merton, R. K., Fiske, M., & Kendall, P. L. (1990). *The focused interview: A manual of problems and procedures* (second edition). New York: The Free Press. (Original edition published in 1956)

Moody, H. R., & Carroll, D. (1997). *The five stages of the soul.* New York: Anchor.

Myerhoff, B. (1980). *Number our days.* New York: Touchstone.

Neugarten, B. (1963). Personality and the aging process. In R. H. Williams, C. Tibbitts, & W. Donahue (Eds.), *Processes of aging: Social and psychological perspectives* (pp. 321–334). New York: Atherton.

O'Nan, S. (2000). *The circus fire.* New York: Doubleday.

Putnam, R. (2000). *Bowling alone: The collapse and revival of American community.* New York: Simon and Schuster.

Reinharz, S. (1992). *Feminist methods in social research.* New York: Oxford University Press.

Riley, M. W., & Foner, A. (1968). *Aging and society: Volume one. An inventory of research findings.* New York: Russell Sage Foundation.

Riley, M. W., Johnson, M., & Foner, A. (1972). *Aging and society: Volume three. A sociology of age stratification.* New York: Russell Sage Foundation.

Rizzuto, A.-M. (1993). Exploring sacred landscapes. In M. L. Randour (Ed.), *Exploring sacred landscapes: Religious and spiritual experiences in psychotherapy* (pp. 16–33). New York: Columbia University Press.

Roof, W. C. (1993). *A generation of seekers: The spiritual journeys of the baby boom generation.* San Francisco: HarperSanFrancisco.

Roof, W. C. (1999). *Spiritual marketplace: Baby-boomers and the remaking of American religion.* New Jersey: Princeton University Press.

Ryder, N. B. (1965). The cohort as a concept in the study of social change. *American Sociological Review, 30,* 843–866.

Savishinsky, J. S. (1991). *The ends of time: Life and work in a nursing home.* New York: Bergin and Garvey.

Schutz, A. (1970). *On phenomenology and social relations* (H. R. Wagner, Ed.). Chicago: University of Chicago Press.

Sexton, A. (1975). *The awful rowing toward God.* Boston: Houghton Mifflin.

Shield, R. R. (1988). *Uneasy endings: Daily life in a nursing home.* Ithaca: Cornell University Press.

Simmel, G. (1971). *On individuality and social forms* (D. Levine, Ed.). Chicago: University of Chicago Press.

Stark, R., & Finke, R. (2000). *Acts of faith.* Berkeley: University of California Press.

Steinsaltz, A. (1988). *The long shorter way* (Y. Hanegbi, Ed. and Trans.). Northvale, NJ: Jason Aronson.

Strauss, A. L. (1959). *Mirrors and masks: The search for identity.* Glencoe, IL: The Free Press.

Sullivan, H. S. (1954). *The psychiatric interview* (H. S. Perry & M. L. Gawel, Eds.). New York: W. W. Norton.

Sumner, W. G. (1940). *Folkways: A study of the sociological importance of usages, manners, customs, mores, and morals.* New York: The New American Library. (Original work published in 1906)

Thomas, L. E., & Eisenhandler, S. A. (1999). *Religion, belief, and spirituality in late life.* New York: Springer.

Thomas, W. I., & Znaniecki, F. (1958). *The Polish peasant in Europe and America.* New York: Dover. (Original work first published in 1918)

Tornstam, L. (1999). Late-life transcendence: A new developmental perspective on aging. In L. E. Thomas & S. A. Eisenhandler (Eds.), *Religion, belief, and spirituality in late life* (pp. 178–202). New York: Springer.

Vaillant, G. E. (1977). *Adaptation to life.* Boston: Little, Brown.

Van Gennep, A. (1960). *The rites of passage* (M. B. Vizedom & G. L. Coffee, Trans.). Chicago: University of Chicago Press. (Original work published in 1908)

Wentroble, D. P. (1999). Pastoral care of problematic Alzheimer's disease and dementia affected residents in long-term care settings. In L. VandeCreek (Ed.), *Spiritual care for persons with dementia: Fundamentals for pastoral care* (pp. 59–76). New York: The Haworth Press.

Wilder, T. (1969). *The bridge of San Luis Rey.* Middlesex, England: Penguin. (Original work published in 1927)

Wrong, D. H. (1961). The oversocialized conception of man in modern sociology. *American Sociological Review, 26,* 183–193.

A Closer Look at Several Steps in the Research Process

The research design for this project on religious behavior and beliefs of older adults is drawn from qualitative methodology and has as its express purpose the depiction of the nature of religious belief and behavior among the old living independently in the community and the old living under various regimes of supervision within long-term care facilities. Appendix A describes in greater detail some of the research procedures that were part of the study and Appendix B summarizes some of the important social characteristics of the 46 elders who were interviewed for the study.

CONTACTING PEOPLE IN THE COMMUNITY AND IN LONG-TERM CARE FACILITIES

Once nominations for the sample had been received (this process was described in chapter 1), I proceeded to contact people to schedule interviews. With respect to older adults in the community, I usually telephoned, and for elders in long-term care I spoke directly with people who had been suggested to me or whom I had observed in my comings and goings within the facility. In some cases, nominators contacted potential interviewees to let them know that I would be calling to talk about the research project and to schedule an appointment.

During my initial phone call or face-to-face contact with the prospective interviewee, I introduced myself and reviewed the purpose of the study as well as the general approach and topics to be covered in the interview. Discussion about the informed consent statement was also part of the first contact I made with candidates for the study. I provided my e-mail address and home and office phone numbers during these initial discussions. Interviews were typically scheduled during the first contact, though for 10 people the first contact or call was actually the second or third phone call because I had left messages previously on their voice mail or message machines. In three cases, people called me back before I had the opportunity to make a second call to them.

Most people had some questions about the amount of time required for the interview. Like all Americans, older adults are busy people with fairly full schedules. Sometimes there were queries about the setting for the interview, who else might be there, or length, and some asked about the general topics (religion and life experiences). During these initial phone conversations and face-to-face chats, a number of people wondered aloud if they had the depth of knowledge to comment extensively about religion. This kind of "testing" response with the accompanying use of disclaimers frequently occurs when people are asked to participate in face-to-face interviews, and is to a considerable degree, a situational response to concerns they have about passing muster and preserving their identity. I assured individuals that the interview was not a test of them or of their understanding of religion. Instead the interview was planned to be a conversation about their lives and experience—topics that made them the best experts I could find. After all, who could be a better source about their own experiences and lives? A few wits had clever responses to that rhetorical question, but people understood the message that the interview was not any sort of test. A handful of people asked me to call back after they had given some thought to the request, but most scheduled the interviews by the close of the first person-to-person chat or telephone call.

The only person in the sample of 46 to call back with a follow-up question about the interview after scheduling an interview, had developed a concern that I might be selling books. After acknowledging some of the unscrupulous ways that older adults were frequently targeted by people selling products, I restated the purpose for the interview—to complete a research project. The outcome of the research would lead to publication of articles and a book, but I would not be selling books or any other products during the interview. With that said, the person agreed to participate. It was a very good question to raise given the merchandising appeals and fraudulent propositions that older adults frequently receive.

This interchange occurred a bit past the midpoint of the interview phase of the study and it gave me the chance to think about any action I might have taken in the research process to create such a misunderstanding. One possible explanation came to mind. Along with a tape recorder and the usual pen and paper accoutrements of research, I always carried with me to each interview a copy of the most recent book a colleague and I had published. Ordinarily I mentioned the book after the close of the formal interview when the discussion turned to questions the interviewee might have about the research or with regard to the next steps in the project. After discussing how many more inter- views would be conducted, and how the information was likely to be used for analysis, I showed the book to interviewees so they could see a tangible outcome from other research studies. Perhaps the meaning of the book had been confused as interviewees talked to others they knew about their participation in the study, or perhaps this was an anomaly, a specific concern from one person. But it seemed as though this innocent or informative act of bringing a book with me might be the culprit. I considered leaving the book behind during future interviews. However, all other interviewees had enjoyed seeing the book and had understood that it was presented as an example of what really happened to all of the words and material collected. So I decided to keep the book in my field research and interviewing toolkit and to see if the issue came up again. It did not. This development was a good example of the fact that the symbolic meaning of items is not uniformly understood, and an even stronger reminder of how important it is for the researcher and the interviewee to share thoughts as a research project progresses.

In a slightly different vein, but still related to sharing thoughts, after the study had ended, a half-dozen people provided additional informa- tion about points they had discussed by mailing copies of letters and other written documents to me. During four of the interviews, people provided additional materials about their lives. As the study drew to its conclusion, a fragment of conversation was overheard by someone working in a community agency located in a town where interviews were gathered. The conversational fragment that was reported to me had to do with someone talking about an interview recently held with a professor doing a study, and that "no, she was not selling books, she was trying to learn more in order to write a new book."

CHARACTERISTICS OF THE LONG-TERM CARE FACILITIES

Selected characteristics of facilities presented in Table A1 are taken from the state-by-state and within-state data compiled by the Health

TABLE A1   Characteristics of Long-Term Care Facilities in Study

Name	County/ Location	Bed Count	Ownership	Hospital	Chain
Chelsea Court	Hartford	200	Religious	No	Yes
Chestnut Grove*	New Haven	100	For profit	No	Yes
Daphne Lane	New Haven	100	Religious	No	No
Ivy Corner	Hartford	300	Religious	Yes	No
Maple Way	New Haven	100	For profit	No	No
White Pines	Hartford	100	Nonprofit	Yes	No

*Chestnut Grove is a long-term care facility where participant observation was completed for the study. Formal interviews were not conducted at Chestnut Grove.

Care Finance Administration (HCFA) from routine reports submitted by nursing homes or long-term care facilities. The variables or characteristics provided in this form of assessment are quite limited in scope, however, the data permit some comparisons among and between institutions and give a general sense of what the institutions are like and the degree to which they vary by a set of uniform criteria over a narrow range of dimensions. The institutional profiles outlined above in Table A1 are for the six long-term care facilities in this study. The facilities are listed alphabetically by pseudonyms used for the study and by their actual county location. The information for the facilities was valid for the interview phase of the study (1999–2000). In order to protect the confidentiality of the institutions, I have rounded the bed counts. Thus, the bed count is an approximate one not exact one. Data on nursing homes is readily available online from the Health Care Finance Administration (HCFA) and is updated periodically. The data presented in Table A1 were accessed from this online address: www.medicare.gov/ NHCompare.

Entrée to Institutions

Though I very much doubt that older adults within long-term care institutions reflect on the range and depth of restricted interaction and the generally benign yet unambiguously bureaucratic ethos that shapes patterns of daily life within these settings, it was a surprise of sorts for me as a dyed-in-the-wool community or noninstitutional researcher to discover that each facility had a different way of working with social scientific research and researchers and accordingly a different stance with respect to the resident's rights in this setting. The one item of agreement across institutions was that some assent or permission, ranging from an institutional awareness of the fact that the researcher was within the facility to a full blown IRB review of their own, was a necessary first step to talking with older adults who lived on the premises. This struck me as paternalistic and at odds with the thrust of much gerontological thinking and research in the past quarter of a century that has consistently underscored the autonomy and abilities of older adults. Notwithstanding this general emphasis on combating ageism from the combined disciplines of gerontology, one only has to cross the threshold into long-term care to discover that older adults here are often thought to be in need of "protection" for their own good. This paternalistic stance toward residents is codified in federal regulations that identify the elderly as members of "protected classes." Much of the institutional outlook seems related to those regulations.

Certainly no one quarrels with providing adequate protections for vulnerable adults, but older adults apparently become vulnerable by a definitional standard that presumes age and residential status are the best criteria for the label. One outcome of this assigned definitional dependency is that research, particularly social research by independent researchers, appears to be more difficult to pursue as scientific or even humanistic inquiry. On balance, as an academic or outside researcher, I was welcome and eventually able to interview people within each institution. Each institution was officially receptive to the study. However, access to the premises to conduct interviews was very difficult in one setting, about what I expected in three settings, and open in two settings.

HOW ELDERS IN LONG-TERM CARE WERE SELECTED AS PARTICIPANTS

Having acquired permission to interview and to cross the threshold into long-term care settings, how did I choose people to interview in the long-term settings? The dilemma of selection is always a feature of social science methodology and methods, and it has direct implications for specific forms of predictive statements. Without delving into lengthy exposition about selection, suffice it to say that it is difficult to select people for interviews in long-term settings without some leads and suggestions from nominators, here, the staff within the facility. To reiterate a point expressed earlier, I found that once I was across the threshold into the long-term care facility, staff members were concerned about helping me find possible interviewees who would be physically and mentally capable of completing an interview and in finding people who might also be comfortable with the experience of talking at length with someone they had never met before and would likely not meet again. Both of these struck me as reasonable criteria that simultaneously acknowledged legitimate rights of the older adult and the purpose of the research project.

Unlike the stiff protectiveness that colored the institutional face of some initial contacts with long-term care administrative staff, the specific discussions of who might be willing and able to talk with me about life events and religion as well as other beliefs, were conversations laced with open possibilities and wide-ranging suggestions about who might like to talk and the various kinds of backgrounds that some staff members had learned about in caring for and working with elderly individuals. Individual staff members were committed to assisting the researcher and with assisting the resident by identifying nominees who might be able and receptive to the research. Moreover, the staff members at this level were so helpful that ultimately I ended up with more leads to pursue for long-term care interviewees than I could actually follow up on in the study. This sensitivity to resident and researcher was a welcome contrast to some of the reluctance that was part of initial contacts with other levels of staff within the facilities.

Such recommendations generated a "yield" problem in that I obtained more names than I could interview. In one facility I explained to an interviewee's roommate, at length and in what was ultimately an unsatisfying way to him and me, that as much as I would like to I could not interview him. I recognized that I might miss his ideas and insights, but in terms of the pressure of time, I could only talk with people who had already agreed to be interviewed. The interviewee's roommate gradually accepted this statement. But it is tough, even for a seasoned field researcher, to be in the position of turning down volunteers, particularly in long-term care facilities where people often look forward to additional interaction. In two long-term care facilities, word of mouth generated some interest among others in the prospect of being interviewed. That had not been the case for the community-dwelling elders, perhaps because I did not use a central point or single organization to develop leads for interviews. In some previous studies, I used senior centers or other age-based groups or programs to assist with offering initial leads for interviewees from which a larger snowball sample emerged.

Accordingly, people chosen as interviewees in the long-term care settings like those in the community sample were nominated by others. The difference was that for long-term care settings most nominees were named by various staff members from the institutions. Two people in long-term care were interviewed based on a nomination from one community dwelling older adult who had been interviewed earlier in the project. With respect to the institutional settings, one interviewee from an institution nominated another person for an interview. In the community sample, two participants nominated other prospects who were interviewed later in the study. Thus, a few participants in the study were part of a snowball sample based on nomination by others.

It is germane to point out that in three institutions where interviews were conducted, I also observed daily activities and use of space by accompanying people (staff members or volunteers) during their usual rounds or series of interactions with older adults in the facility. I spent some time on my own within these facilities, but my participant observation was both observation and an undisguised or visible shadowing; that is, I provided an extra set of hands and legs to various people as they worked with older adults. In the course of conducting interviews and as part of my role as an observer, I was asked to do several tasks which brought me rather naturally into the interactions and activities that involved a variety of social actors and areas or places within the institution. This was advantageous for the research project because it allowed me to glimpse other areas of daily life within the institution and added depth to my firsthand understanding of the kinds of possible routes for the practice of faith and religiosity within the institutions. There are boundaries within institutions to the individual's ability and willingness to pursue or follow some religious behaviors. These structural limitations on the expression of faith were on a par with the limitations some interviewees faced from health problems. Poor health or the inability to balance and cope with physical and socioemotional aspects of health and aging brought the people I interviewed into the institution, and once there, exercising and practicing one's faith and religion were almost equally shaped by the person's health status as well as the presence of institutional constraints. The structural constraints I observed were systemic rather than personal in that they did not appear to be the result of any individual's motivation or behavior toward the resident or interviewee. The constraints were, as was discussed in chapter 6, sociological features of the social organization of the institution. Selected characteristics of these facilities are presented in Appendix A, Table A1.

OTHER SELECTION ISSUES: REFUSALS AND "VOLUNTEERS"

For the entire group the refusal rate, the number of people who were asked to participate and declined the interview, was scant. There was one refusal from a person in the community dwelling sample and none from the long-term care sample. The sole refusal came from a person who had initially agreed to an interview. She talked with me later to tell me she had reconsidered and wished to forgo it. She explained that it would be difficult to "put my beliefs about God into words." I also spent some time at a senior center talking with a group of billiard players, hoping from this contact to develop a few leads for interviews from them. In this instance, prospective interviewees were not forthcoming either as volunteers for an interview or as sources of nominees.

In an opposite vein, several older adults in the community, eight, approached me to "volunteer" for the study and the interview. They talked with me about their wish to be interviewed. These eight volunteers had to be turned down as participants because I was too close to them in a number of important ways. That degree of closeness was, I thought, a likely and substantial source for bias in interpretation and analysis of the interviews.

INTERVIEWS AND THE SETTINGS FOR INTERVIEWS

Interviews typically lasted from 90 minutes to 120 minutes. The shortest interview was 45 minutes; the longest was well over 3 1/2 hours. Both of these were community interviews. In general, the long-term care interviews were shorter, though a handful of these were also fairly long, approaching the 2 hour mark. With two exceptions (living room of the researcher and a small reading room of a public library), interviews with the community elders were held in the homes or personal living space of the interviewee. With two exceptions, there was no other person in the room when the researcher and interviewee were talking. In one instance, a translator known to both parties was part of the interview. In the second instance, a spouse was contributing actively and met the social parameters for the study, so I asked the spouse to participate and conducted two interviews. All other interviews with married couples were held separately and privately. In terms of logistics, these interviews were, with one exception, held in time periods that were back-to-back, typically with a break between the separate interviews.

In long-term care settings the interview setting was subject to a number of situational factors. Nearly all of the interviews were conducted in private, but the settings varied slightly from the person's living space to quiet, small rooms in various parts of five facilities. In one long-term care setting, multiuse space was provided for one of the interviews. However, just as we were ready to begin, it was clear that the interviewee was not quite comfortable (apparently one of the room's other uses was for memorial services). Together we found table and chairs in an unoccupied computer room and proceeded to use that space for our conversation.

THE INTERVIEW GUIDE

Questions in the interview protocol were open-ended and the interview was semi-structured or focused (Merton, Fiske, & Kendall, 1990). Uniform phrasing was used for some sets of questions, particularly those directed to social background and life in childhood and early adulthood. In general, there was a chronological and biographical order to the interview questions, but there were also many opportunities to follow up with questions that illuminated the unique characteristics of individuals and their life stories. At times topics arose spontaneously and unexpectedly. These topics were ones pursued in the interview, and once discussed, we returned to the general time order of the protocol. About one-quarter of the protocol asked for information about social background and for comments or retrospective accounts of what life was like during childhood and young adulthood. The remaining questions, about three-quarters of the protocol, asked the interviewee about various aspects of religious and spiritual beliefs and behaviors. People were asked to recall and describe selected aspects of their childhood and adulthood and to tell me about their daily life today and the religious, spiritual, or other beliefs that have meaning for them.

The guide was used as exactly that, a guide. There was not a rigid format to the interview though particular comparative and purposive information was sought from all interviewees (such as religious affiliation of parents, and the denominational background of the person across his or her life). This information also provided a way to reflect upon and weigh the homogeneity or variability within the group. A copy of some of the questions from the interview schedule is included in this appendix. There was no significant adjustment of language, order, or subject matter of questions or the protocol overall as I interviewed elders in long-term care facilities.

Selected Questions from the Interview Guide

Section A of the guide included several questions about family background and what life was like for the person when she or he was growing up. Section A also included a few questions about the family life and social experiences of early to middle adulthood. Religion often came up spontaneously in discussion and responses to other questions in Section A. However, Section B contained the specific questions on religion.

Selected questions from Section B are reproduced here. Questions about religious identification, membership, attendance, involvement, financial support, and other similar formal measures of religiosity were asked but are not included here. The numbers of individual questions do not reflect the precise order of questions in the guide, but they are accurate chronological markers of the general flow and order of topics and questions in the guide. Though I expected some elders to make use of the word spirituality (and it was listed parenthetically in the interview guide wherever I used the word religion), people in the study used the words religion and faith to describe their experiences as related to the sacred and to the communities of believers surrounding the sacred. Also, there were some questions about mobility and services that were more germane to elders in long-term care facilities than to other elders.

Section C of the guide, the closing, is not reproduced here. It contained a handful of questions about faith—the person's sense of how she or he saw religious congregations changing, ideas and beliefs changing, and their own practice continuing or changing. The Governor of Minnesota, Jesse Ventura's, widely circulated quotation about religion's appeal as directed to people who were "weak-minded" was used in one of the questions in Section C. The interview concluded with comments and observations from the participant and with a summary from the interviewer of where the project was going and how the information gathered in the study would disclose patterns of commonality and of difference among elders on religious and social dimensions.

Selected Questions from Section B of the Interview Guide for the Study

NOW I'D LIKE TO ASK YOU SOME QUESTIONS ABOUT RELIGIOUS AND SPIRITUAL EXPERIENCES OVER THE COURSE OF YOUR LIFE. I'LL BE ASKING YOU ABOUT YOUR LIFE TODAY BUT I'LL BEGIN WITH SOME QUESTIONS ABOUT GROWING UP.

1. When you were growing up, in what religion (religious tradition) were you raised?
2. Who taught you the basics of your religion (faith)?
    Probes and comments.
3. What is the first important religious experience you recall?
4. What did religion (faith) mean to you back then?
5. Have you changed your religion during your lifetime?
    Can you tell me more about the change? Probes for occasion(s); people involved, length of time in this faith; reasons for changes.
5. Have your religious (spiritual) beliefs changed over the course of your lifetime?
6. What kinds of religious (spiritual) experiences have been important to you? [Which were ones you did not want to miss, ones you looked forward to? Which could you have skipped or missed?]
7. During your life were there particular people who played significant roles in your religious (spiritual) experience?
8. Over your lifetime were there instances where you sacrificed something in order to maintain your religious beliefs or to practice your religion (faith)?
9. Were there instances when you changed your personal views or social behavior because your religious beliefs provided you with guidance?
10. Thinking about your religious experience today, in what ways does your religion matter to you?

11. I'd like you to think about a typical day of activities. What kinds of acts and activities do you engage in that you think of as religious (spiritual)?

12. I'd like you to think about a typical week of activities. What kinds of acts and activities do you engage in that you think of as religious (spiritual)?

13. During the past three months (June–August 1999 for initial interviewees, adjusted as time progressed and study continued) have there been special occasions that you participated in that you would think of as religious (spiritual)?

14. What kinds of things do you do daily to keep your religious (spiritual) beliefs alive?

15. What kinds of things do you do weekly to keep your religious (spiritual) beliefs alive?

16. What kinds of things do you do over the course of a year to keep your religious (spiritual) beliefs alive?

17. Have you gone through dry periods (droughts) in your religious (spiritual) life?

18. Have you gone through periods of questioning religious (spiritual) beliefs?

19. When I use the term religious or spiritual, do particular people come to mind?

20. Are there people you look up to or seek out to talk to because they are religious or spiritual?

21. Many people say that belonging to an organized religious group is the best way to define someone as religious or spiritual. What do you think about that?

22. Some people say that one feature of religious maturity or heightened spirituality is a greater concern for others (not merely your family and friends). What do you think?

22A. Have you noticed that you have a greater concern for others today than you did when you were younger? [A recent example that virtually everyone was aware of from the Fall of 1999 was the earthquake in Turkey. I used this as a reference point in many interviews. People often moved from that particular instance to other examples that they wished to talk about.]

23. Some people say that one feature of religious engagement, especially a heightened awareness of religion (spirituality), is a direct sense of divine presence in one's life.
    Have you experienced what you thought was the direct presence of God (or a divine force) in your life?

24.   In what ways do you think you have transmitted (passed on) your religious (spiritual) beliefs to others?
       Probes and nested questions about adult children, nieces and nephews, grandchildren, others.

25.   Is there anything you'd like to change about your religious (spiritual) life?

25A.   Probes for what and how to change.

26.   When you think of all the different people and ideas and activities that matter in your life today, where would you place religion (spirituality)?
       [After several people suggested that this was like creating a top 10 list, I changed the wording to elicit the rank of religion in the top 10 of the person's list of interests and activities]. The question then became: If you stop to think of 10 of the most important activities that matter to you these days, where would you place religion?
       Probes and comments.

Some Social Characteristics
of the Sample

Highlights of the sample were discussed in Chapter 1. Appendix B provides further discussion of some important social characteristics of the group as a whole (46) and separately with respect to those residing in the community (31) and those residing in long-term care (15). Table B1 presents the participants in the study by place of residence and by residential status (community or long-term care).

SELECTED SOCIAL CHARACTERISTICS
OF THE SAMPLE

Tables B2 and B3 reflect the age and sex distributions for community-dwelling and long-term care interviewees.

The mean age for community-dwelling men was 80, for women it was 76. For men and women combined, the mean age was 77 with a mode at 74 and a median of 78. The age range in the community-dwelling sample was 60–93.

The mean age for men residing in long-term care settings was 77, for women it was 86. For men and women combined, the mean age was 83 and the mode and median ages were 79. The age range was 73–96.

Religious identification and active involvement were discussed in chapter 1. Everyone interviewed for the study had a clear religious identification that for the most part, as noted earlier in chapters 1 and 2, stemmed from parental ascription and childhood socialization. For the study as a whole, religious identification was as follows: Roman Catholics, 21; Protestants, 18; Jews, 7. Table B4 presents religious identification by residential status.

**TABLE B1   Participants in the Study
Listed Alphabetically by Place of Residence and First Name***

Residents of Long-Term Care Facilities	
Facility and Town (pseudonyms)	Interviewee (pseudonym)
Chelsea Court, Deer Park	Anne
	Ellen
	James
	Marie
Daphne Lane, Stowe Landing	Barbara
	Douglas
	Patrick
	Val
Ivy Corner, Deer Park	Arthur
	Joan
	Sarah
Maple Way, Millerville	Ruth
White Pines, Farmvale	Alice
	Carol
	Margaret

Community-Dwelling Participants		
Town (pseudonym)	Interviewee (pseudonym)	Age
Beecher Bend	Stephen	85
Coltville	Gwen	80
	Wanda	83
Crandall Point	Eugene	82
	Nora	77
Ellaburg	Andrew	92
	Lydia	89
Laurelford	Beth	71
	Clara	90
	Donna	62
	Edward	60
	Gail	63
	Hank	80
	Larry	74
	Jean	72
	Marilyn	78
	Martha	74
	Pauline	87
	Phillip	93
	Robert	85
	Sally	79

(continued)

TABLE B1   *(continued)*

Community-Dwelling Participants		
Town (pseudonym)	Interviewee (pseudonym)	Age
Ledgeton	Julia	75
Millerville	Alex	76
	Libby	74
	Lucy	76
	Rose	68
Samuelson	Grace	61
	Peter	79
	Walter	70
	Victoria	90
Twainbury	Maxine	77

*Ages are not listed for long-term care participants in order to preserve the privacy of individuals in such a small subset.

TABLE B2   Age and Sex Distribution for Community-Dwelling Residents

Age	Female	Male	Total
60–64	3	1	4
65–74	5	2	7
75–84	8	4	12
85+	4	4	8
Total	20	11	31

TABLE B3   Age and Sex Distribution for Long-Term Care Residents

Age	Female	Male	Total
60–64	0	0	0
65–74	0	2	2
75–84	6	1	7
85+	5	1	6
Total	11	4	15

TABLE B4   Religious Identification by Kind of Residence

Residence	Roman Catholic	Protestant	Jewish	Total
Community	13	15	3	31
Long-term care	8	3	4	15
Total	21	18	7	46

Religious identification does not automatically translate into membership in an actual congregation. This was especially true for Roman Catholic elders in this study. Roman Catholics were slightly less likely to have an active involvement in formal worship than either Protestant or Jewish older adults. With respect to the long-term care residents, no one spoke of belonging (even in the facilities that had dedicated space for worship) to the congregation on site; instead they spoke of belonging to the congregations they had been members of before moving into the facility.

In other words, everyone had a religious affiliation, and nearly all were actively engaged in private, personal religious behavior, but some did not participate regularly in formal worship. Moreover, a few were not members of a congregation nor did they participate in formal worship on a regular basis. The number of active participants in formal, religious services is displayed in Table B5.

MARITAL STATUS, EDUCATION, FINANCES

With respect to marital status in the total group, 18 were widowed, 17 were married (among the 17 in the married category are 10 people or

TABLE B5   Active Religious Participation by Kind of Residence

Residence	Roman Catholic	Protestant	Jewish	Total
Community	8	13	3	24
Long-term care	7	2	1	10
Total	15	15	4	34

5 couples who are married), 8 were single (had never married), and 3 were divorced or separated. In the community-dwelling sample, 18 people lived with others and 13 lived alone. In the long-term care sample, 5 people lived alone; that is, they had private rooms, and 10 shared a room with one other person, a roommate who in one instance was a spouse. With respect to other social characteristics, the sample included people who had completed the equivalent of junior high school to those who had completed graduate school (the highest level was the master's degree).

The relationships among age, sex, and education were not entirely straightforward in this sample as the highest levels of education were most often associated with women rather than men, and the oldest rather than the youngest older adults. The typical member of the sample had completed or graduated from high school. Related to the level of educational attainment, a majority of the sample described themselves as "having enough money to provide for the basics of living and to do some of the things I enjoy."

At either extreme of the financial continuum, there were about equal numbers of people: a handful possessed extensive financial security, and alternatively, a handful faced serious financial difficulty. Not all of those facing some financial difficulty were residents of long-term care, although many residents of long-term care described themselves as having already faced and adapted to stringent financial constraints if not outright hardship. Most people termed their financial position as "adequate" in terms of their life experiences and some added "for people my age." It is important to recognize that the reference groups for these general assessments of social standing (sufficient income, financial security, and even health status) were based on comparisons with "others my age," not with cohorts of younger people. My impression is that others my age means people in the same decade (with the person's age operating as the midpoint of that decade).

The greatest concern expressed by community-dwelling elderly was related to finances. This concern, one that is documented in other research studies, was found in the statement that "I may outlive my money." Many in the long-term sample spoke of having already "over-spent" their personal financial resources, an oblique but telling remark about the fact that they were recipients of subsidized care. In the sample as a whole, only a small number of people were currently employed (earning wages). In this group the number of hours worked weekly varied widely with three people in the 30–40 hour range that is frequently used to define full-time participation in the labor force.

HEALTH

The general health of the sample as evaluated from questions and direct observation of movement, posture, voice, hearing, and attentiveness to items in the interview, was at least satisfactory across the group. For a smaller number, general health was good to very good when compared with others their age. In both groups, the community-dwelling and the long-term care residents, chronic health problems were widely mentioned as part of the individual's experience. Some described a range of serious, medical conditions that were ongoing, but "manageable," as one person phrased it. Two people had serious, life-threatening illnesses.

Moreover, in the long-term care group, everyone had at least one, and typically more than one, ongoing health problem that resulted in both debilitating and comprehensive individual frailty. Most, but not every person in the long-term care sample used assistive technology, from hearing aids to various kinds of canes, walkers, or wheelchairs. Similarly most were unable to be mobile (ambulatory) without consistent reliance upon mechanical or human assistance.

On the whole, the community-dwelling sample possessed a greater degree of physical mobility as evidenced in walking without assistive technology, steadier gaits, wider range of body motion, higher levels of physical energy, as well as in their ability to drive automobiles. No one interviewed in the long-term care settings continued to drive as contrasted with the community sample where there were less than a handful of non-drivers. Among the community-dwelling group, 20 people had devised and regularly used some adaptive strategies for driving (e.g., not driving at night, limiting their range to immediate community, avoiding limited access highways, driving at off-peak times, driving with a companion). In comparison, the long-term sample was more tightly bound to the facility. They were able to get about outside the facility with group transportation, rides from family and friends, and in one case, walking. However, such excursions were rare. Most were much less able to get about in the larger social world and many were confined to moving about in the institution or in their immediate surroundings.

Though no one in the sample had perfect health, most had adapted and coped satisfactorily with various health problems. The long-term care sample was on the whole much more frail physically than were the community-dwelling elders. With respect to general indicators of mental health, such as an orientation of time, to the setting, and to the interview, nearly everyone was able to respond in a socially appropriate fashion. This is unsurprising because nominators were inclined to nominate people who were cognitively and socially capable of thinking about questions and answering them. Two people did have some difficulty in staying within the situational framework of the interview, and one of these two experienced great difficulty in keeping within the boundaries of social time and within the subject matter of the interview. Indeed, the two older adults with tangible deficits in this area were from the community sample.

In different ways and with different emphases, all of those interviewed had experienced measures of happiness and sadness, and the gains and losses that are part of living and of the process of growing old. People described their lives as good, not perfect, and most but not everyone had some plans, hopes, and dreams for the future. The focus of those dreams and plans was narrow, but it was described and in some instances served to provide meaning and motivation for people to carry on with life itself. In the long-term care sample these plans were more profoundly limited by a lack of mobility and greater frailty as well as serious illness among the elders. There was a clear sense that people residing in long-term care facilities understood that their future was not as open to possibility as it once had been. The future had narrowed and they were aware of that change, but even in the most serious cases of discouraged individuals with serious health problems, the idea of a future had not been entirely foreclosed. In long-term care settings among interviewees who participated in social and devotional activities, I observed a wide range of affect or expressive behavior during those interactions, much more than I discerned in their behavior during other kinds of social interaction in the facility.

PLACE AND LIVING ARRANGEMENTS

Geographically the study covered the northwest corner of Connecticut to the central part of the state, or the upper northwest to mid-state quadrant. If the state is divided into four roughly equal quadrants using the city of Middletown as an approximate midpoint, people interviewed are found in the northwest-central quadrant. All participants in the study resided in the following Connecticut towns and cities: Avon, Bristol, Canaan, Hartford, Meriden, Plainville, Sharon, Simsbury, South Windsor, Southington, Waterbury, and West Hartford. Pseudonyms were assigned to these communities. These 12 communities are found in three (Hartford, Litchfield, and New Haven) of Connecticut's eight counties and include rural villages, small towns, suburbs, and large cities. The state of Connecticut has a total of 169 cities and towns. More than 1,800 miles were logged in during the interviewing and observational portions of the study.

As was discussed in chapter 1, this sample had long and deep residential roots in the state and in the greater New England region. This was also true for most of the 15 elders who lived in long-term care facilities; however, the situation with regard to the length of residency in these specific long-term care settings was somewhat different. Although there were three people who had lived in long-term care facilities for 8 to 10 years, some of those years had been spent in residence at the same site but in a different section of the facility. They had formerly lived in an area of the facility that was designed for "independent living" and had moved into a section that provided greater supportive services. At least three members of the community-dwelling sample had other housing and living arrangements available to them in warmer climes during the Connecticut winter, but the majority were year-round residents of the state. This solid residential stability may be the most important structural variable to influence the long-lived salience of religion found among this group of 46 elders.

The type of housing found among those in the community-dwelling sample varied from some elders who resided in publicly funded housing projects (subsidized apartments) to those in private apartments in homes (e.g., renting part of a two-family house), to those who rented units in relatively large, private apartment complexes, to ownership of a private residence in a "gated" community. The majority of elders owned their own homes—single-family detached houses. Two people owned condominiums as their primary residences and one person had separate premises within a single family home shared with family members. Though many kinds of retirement communities may be found within this geographical quadrant of the state, no one in the study resided in such a community. Three of the six long-term care facilities had multi-levels of residential arrangements and health care including units for "independent living." Two elders in the long-term care sample resided in such units, and received some kinds of support for household tasks. Thirteen others had residential arrangements that were directly linked to more extensive medical and social support for daily life.

A SENSE OF BELONGING AND CONNECTEDNESS

In terms of immediate family, other than spouses or other family members (siblings, adult children) who shared living space, nearly everyone had at least one family member or close friend within a half-hour's drive. Among community-dwelling elders, 18 lived with others and 13 lived alone. Among the long-term care elders, 10 lived with others and 5 lived alone. Even among those elders who were the poorest in this study, the physical condition of housing was adequate and most were satisfied with their housing arrangements. However, all people interviewed voiced concerns about transportation and expressed a range of concerns about health care, from cost to quality to specific treatment for health problems.

More problematic for some older adults in the community and for most in long-term care was the lack of regular interaction with a larger set of people outside of those in their immediate environment. Most elders had one or two friends or family members with whom they shared continuing, meaningful, and satisfactory interaction, but as one person said, "sometimes, Susan, I go for days without talking to anyone personally [face-to-face]." Social isolation is not a prominent feature or typical of those in the study, but when it was part of a person's life, it exerted a profound influence and people were fully aware of it as part of their life. Five people, three in long-term care and two in the community, could be described as being utterly alone (having only sporadic and infrequent face-to-face interaction with someone they'd like to talk with). Three of these five had some formal family and friendship ties within a relatively close commute.

Index